Great Words of the Bible

Prescriptions for Spiritual Health

Great Words of the Bible

Prescriptions for Spiritual Health

Dr. Theodore B. Kalivoda
Professor Emeritus

Pleasant Word

Packaged by Pleasant Word, PO Box 428, Enumclaw, WA 98022. The views expressed or implied in this work do not necessarily reflect those of Pleasant Word. The author(s) is ultimately responsible for the design, content and editorial accuracy of this work.

ISBN 1-4141-0055-8
Library of Congress Catalog Card Number: 2003113362

Contents

Author's Note

I have read many Christian-oriented books in which the authors sounded like spiritual giants who had conquered all the issues they were addressing. It was as if they were saying they had grown beyond the problems and therefore knew what to prescribe for their readers. Whether that was their intent, I cannot say. As far as this writing is concerned, I do not wish to convey my total personal victory over the issues which you are about to read. I must confess that on several occasions I put down the pen out of respect for the idea of writing on anything, especially Christian living, unless I could say I was practicing what I preached. Do I have the right, I asked myself, to talk about spiritual living when so often I lose sight of it in my own life? But at the same time I realize that, like everyone else, I am not immune from stumbling.

We learn from the Lord little by little, probably because, for some reason or other, we are unable to perceive in one instant all the characteristics he would have us apply to our lives. So I write about what God has taught me in bits and pieces. At the same time, I acknowledge my frailties, saying with the apostle Paul, "Not that I have already obtained all this, or have already been made perfect, but I press on" (Phil. 3:12).

May this book be of help in your spiritual quest to better understand God's intent for you. I see the contents as God's prescriptions for our spiritual health.

Preface

The Bible contains many words we can identify as "great." Undoubtedly the list varies in accord with the impact certain words have on an individual. I have chosen three—*grace, faith* and *love*—which I believe encompass many, if not most, traits God considers crucial for spiritual healthy Christians.

The three words interconnect and support each other. One without the others would be difficult if not impossible to practice. As we understand God's marvelous plan of *grace* for salvation as well as *grace* for daily living, we embrace it by exercising *faith*. Both grace and faith are followed by *love* expressed in the form of intimacy with God and a caring relationship with people. That must have been in the mind of the apostle Paul as he commended believers in Colossae:

> We have heard of your *faith* in Christ Jesus and of the *love* you have for all the saints—the faith and love that spring from the hope that is stored up for you in heaven

> and that you have already heard about in the word of truth, the gospel, that has come to you. All over the world this gospel is bearing fruit and growing, just as it has been doing among you since the day you heard it and understood God's *grace* in all its truth. (emphases mine) (Col. 1:4–6)

Understanding grace, putting faith into practice, and practicing love toward people—ingredients for spiritual growth and fruitfulness. Grace, faith and love—great words of the Bible!

I try to show how we may experience the full impact of those words in daily living. I see them as the scriptural key for unlocking the door to a joyful Christian life. They carry an impact on life to such a degree that they combat the ills befalling us on our Christian journey. Indeed, they represent God's prescriptions for our spiritual health.

We have the prescriptions written out in the Bible. But they will do us little good if left lying around unfilled. They must be activated and their contents internalized. Let's see what God, the great physician, prescribes.

Part I, on Grace, concentrates on God's marvelous initiation of a new covenant through Jesus Christ. Its full provisions often go unrecognized as we mistakenly cling to the error of following rules to put us in good stead with our Creator. Contrasted with self-effort in gaining God's approval, the new covenant sets us free from practices we may have thought were appropriate Christian behavior but in reality create a false sense of spirituality that cripples us from enjoying the benefits of Christianity to the fullest.

Chapter One, *Understanding Grace*, begins with God's instruction for obtaining eternal life. That will be good news to anyone not sure of going to heaven. But it will also be a glorious revelation to those who, although acknowledging salvation, feel it necessary to add certain behavioral requirements as an assist to obtaining God's promise of heaven. Scripture has a lot to say about that. We will see how the Bible clearly distinguishes between our own efforts and those displayed by God through his grace. We will also see the mistakes some first-century Christians made in confusing the two, and the disastrous consequences of those errors. Learning from them will keep us on course for Christian living.

People seem to have a natural inclination to engage in making improvements on God's declarations. The religious leaders of Jesus' time did so by creating new laws on top of God's edicts recorded in their Old Testament scriptures. Those rules were burdensome, and Jesus condemned the whole process of supplementing God's prescribed behaviors with those made by people. But Christians today fare no better, often making demands on fellow believers that Scripture gives them no right to do.

Such legalistic requirements tend to be negatively oriented in the sense that they tell us what we must *not* do, all in the guise of spirituality. I experienced as a young Christian the onslaught of those grace killers. It was to my hurt. I will include personal examples of how that happened with the hope that they be instructional to you.

God's plan for us is to experience his goodness. It is not a design that inhibits us from enjoying our new life in Christ. I will delve into its specifics, which will be to our joy. It will set us free from the bondage of thinking we have to perform to find God's acceptance.

Another aspect of grace, discussed in Chapter 2, *Growing in Grace,* is not a single happening as is salvation. It is tied to a dependency on God as we hearken to the persuasions of his Spirit. In contrast, we are used to doing things ourselves and according to our own designs. We all, at one time or another, fail to take advantage of God's help as we exert self-effort which, when failing to measure up to God's standards, causes feelings of guilt, frustration, and discouragement. Sometimes we even get disgusted with ourselves because we have scriptural knowledge reflecting intellectual understanding but devoid of personal experience. In other words, we may know of the Bible's instruction on close fellowship with God, but with little application. Others may not see us this way, but we do, and it can eventually get us down. Struggling within us are gross feelings of inadequacy and even hypocrisy.

It is important to emphasize that growing in grace is a lifelong process. That is why Peter encouraged us to "grow in grace." Because of human limitations, we never arrive in terms of experiencing grace's full potential. But God tells us how we can hook up to the process and watch it grow. And it will be to our joy.

Accepting grace makes for happy Christians. It sets us free from insecurity, frustration, guilt and feelings of shame. Although through human frailty we err from God's ways from time to time, we understand that those shortcomings do not negate God's acceptance of us. No! It is not merely a matter of acceptance. It is more exact to say it involves profound, divine love. Therein lies the definition of grace—God's goodness in loving us in spite of our faults. So, no more long faces! They are to be replaced with happy ones.

Part II (Chapter 3), on *Faith,* dares not exclude faith relative to salvation. Its main emphasis in this writing, however, is to explore faith in terms of Jesus' reference to a full or abundant life. It reinforces the first word of our analysis—grace. We might say that grace and faith are sisters. Both are integral components of God's prescription for spiritual health.

Faith develops intimacy with God to the extent that we become conscious of and thrive on his personal communication. It also instills an attitude of trust in an omniscient, omnipotent, and omnipresent Lord who is always in control and cognizant of our needs no matter what may befall us. Faith helps us rest in all circumstances, as the psalmist declares,

> My soul finds rest in God alone . . . I will never be shaken. (Ps. 62:1–2)

David found rest in God. However, for us today living in the post-cross era, resting in God becomes even more meaningful as we apply it to faith in Christ and his resulting relationship with us. We acknowledge God's complete acceptance through belief in his son, and we react to life's events believing in God's total control and intimate concern. However, we don't resign to life's circumstances by saying that what happens is meant to be. Faith also calls for approaching a caring heavenly Father for his intervention in all that happens to us. Throughout the Bible, faith, or believing God's declarations, is depicted as a virtue greatly honored by God for lightening our load in daily living. His provision for direct petitioning is a privilege that extends the communication process through prayer.

However, failing to heed biblical instruction on the nature of our prayers, we often experience frustration and disenchantment with the whole process. We will explore this area of faith to better understand how best to approach God in prayer.

Part III, on *Love*, approaches the subject in three distinct ways: love toward God; love toward Christians; and love toward all people. Love is a by-product of grace and faith. Out of gratitude to God for his involvement in our lives, we grow in love toward him and extend that love toward people. In fact, God wishes to use us to demonstrate his love toward others. That is one of his means of revealing himself—working through us for the benefit of other people. It is a beautiful privilege, but at the same time an awesome responsibility.

Chapter 4, *Loving God*, challenges us to grow in love by experiencing communication with God. Communicating makes for closeness, and it is done both by listening and talking to him. His communication with us is shown through his written Word, the Bible, but it also takes other forms as we experience his presence in all of life's circumstances. Our goal is to develop a sensitivity to his communication in order to recognize it as coming from God and to receive it with grateful hearts.

We then talk to him, which allows us to express our hearts on whatever we may be experiencing. That talk goes beyond petitioning; it encompasses praise, thanksgiving, and honoring and glorifying his name, all of which come out of a love relationship with him.

God wills that our love for him extend to loving Christians. Chapter 5 explores ways to do that, one of which, meeting together to render mutual spiritual help, has tended to fall by the wayside. A Christian gathering is often defined solely as a Sunday morning worship service. That "meeting" serves a good purpose for reflecting on God's love for us and our love for him, but it is not designed for growing in love toward one another. Something else must come into play—a commitment to fellow Christians that involves listening to them, encouraging them, and serving them. It is an on-going commitment, not just an occasional or rare encounter. We will explore a means of enhancing that love relationship among Christians through small group fellowships which I call care groups.

Love was Jesus' main emphasis. He showed it by giving himself to people. We too are expected to do the same, but we are uncomfortable with the idea out of uncertainty of its requirements. The direction this mutual spiritual care might take comprises important elements in this writing.

Chapter 6 depicts love expressing itself through our dealings with people in general. What great opportunities exist in a strife-ridden world to exhibit love through humanitarian acts. People, including little children, cry out because of hunger, disease, wars and other disasters. Even in our own localities, needs for help are apparent in a myriad of ways. Generosity, as seen in giving of one's time, labor, and material goods, is the mark of a Christian concerned about those in need.

Christians, however, are not to concern themselves only with charitable acts for helping with physical and material needs. By virtue of our grace relationship with God, we are in a position to practice graciousness in the spiritual realm too. We put love into action as we reflect God's provision of salvation. Some Christians are more skillful than others in this endeavor. Many approach the task badly. The latter experience embarrassment, discomfort and even guilt over their poor performance, oftentimes failing to acknowledge that God uses even their bungling words in positive ways for his glory.

But sharing God's love with others is not only done verbally; it is expressed silently through the way we live. Sometimes the latter has even greater impact than the oral message. However, both form a part of the Christian's witness, which shines God's love with brightness to all the world.

Grace, faith and love—God's prescriptions for spiritual wellness. We learn of them and practice them to experience the wonders of God's ways. This book presents a fresh look at those three great words of the Bible by emphasizing their potential for personal experience above and beyond mere knowledge. It suggests means by which readers can apply those virtues for their joy as well as for the joy of those with whom they come in contact. May you be blessed as you take your journey through grace, faith, and love.

Part 1

- GRACE -

CHAPTER 1

Understanding Grace

"For it is by grace you have been saved, through faith—and this not from yourselves, it is the gift of God—not by works, so that no one can boast."

Ephesians 2:8–9

Grace—a critical word for understanding God's message through Jesus Christ. We don't find it used much in secular speech, maybe because it smacks of the Bible, which many people don't like to talk about. Whenever the word is spoken, however, it often leaves hearers uncertain about its meaning. I find that to be true even among many professing Christians.

The situation is unfortunate because "Grace" is pivotal for understanding and practicing true Christianity. It carries a message of such import that New Testament writers were divinely inspired to refer repeatedly to grace. In fact, they used it 155 times to declare God's critical message to humanity—a pronouncement affecting our eternal destiny as well as our well-being on earth. Whether you are a Christian or are in the process of investigating Christianity, by understanding and claiming grace you will be reminded of God's love and desire for cementing an intimate relationship with you. That intimacy will be for your joy.

Characteristics of Grace

The Greek language speaks of grace as *charis*, meaning beauty and charm. That seems to be reflected in John's gospel as it refers to Jesus being "full of grace and truth" (John 1:14). The life of Jesus was one of true inner beauty. That concept is probably what Paul and Peter were reflecting in their epistles when they greeted believers with "grace be unto you." Paul even ended his writings with a grace blessing: "The grace of the Lord Jesus be with you."

Can you catch the spirit of it? It is as if they were saying, "grace translates into a beautiful life, a restful life, a cheerful life, a giving life, one of security, peace and joy." It is a life that exudes God. Jesus pulled it all together by calling the life he preached an abundant or full life (John 10:10). Grace, then, is goodness, something to be enjoyed. It is foundational for full appreciation of all that God would have for us as we journey in the Christian life.

I hope I have aroused your curiosity so that you are saying, "If grace does that, then I want it."

But let's go further. Another mark of "grace" is that it is something not earned—the exact opposite of self-effort. It begins with faith in the death of Christ the Savior. The meaning of Savior, or rescuer, commands attention; it is associated with salvation, which is a gift and therefore by definition is free (Eph. 2:8–9). Since it is free, it can't be bought or earned, because "free" means a gift without charge. It is connected with Jesus Christ sacrificing himself on our behalf through his cross death to free us from sin and thereby make us acceptable to God the Father. It is incredible! I think you will agree—that act of Jesus is of inestimable value, yet it doesn't cost us one cent.

On several occasions Jesus spoke to his disciples about his upcoming death. But not until after his Crucifixion and Resurrection were they enlightened on the meaning behind it. The Holy Spirit revealed its uniqueness—a sacrifice that makes people righteous before God simply on the basis of their acceptance of it through faith. That was undoubtedly an earthshaking experience for the apostles who, immediately after Jesus' crucifixion, were totally stunned over the loss of their Messiah. They must have been completely confused, probably sharing the thoughts of the men who, on the road leading out of Jerusalem toward Emmaus, unknowingly encountered the risen Jesus. We are told that their faces showed them to be completely downcast as they expressed disappointment over the happenings of the past few days. Their problem was they didn't understand that Jesus was to be a sacrifice in order to make them right with God.

Understanding the sacrificial death of Jesus helps us appreciate grace more fully. It was Jewish custom according to the Mosaic Law to offer repeated sacrifices for sins committed. But with the advent of Christ, God initiated a change so remarkable yet so contrary to human expectations that first century Jews found it hard to believe. It is even so for people today. It has to do with one single act, one that takes the place of all others. But that one act would be unique, entirely different from those preceding it, because it would not be performed by people but by God.

What? God performing a sacrifice? Why? He didn't do anything requiring forgiveness, as did people of the Old

Testament. He can't commit any wrongdoing. He is God! But do you know that the sacrifice he made went far beyond the conventional animal offering? This time it was something unequaled in time—God giving his son, Jesus Christ, in the form of a human body, through crucifixion. Had Jesus tried to explain it to his first century audience he would undoubtedly have gotten the response: "What? The Messiah, God himself, dying for us? Impossible! Incomprehensible!" Likely they would have told him to get lost, or that he deserved to die for lying. And that is precisely what happened a few years later. But it wasn't because of a lie, but because of fulfillment of prophecy given hundreds of years earlier (Isa. 53) (Ps. 22:1–18). They rejected him as their Savior.

Unfortunately, unbelief is the stance of many today, even though the Bible clearly spells out God's provision for forgiveness under the rubric of grace. The old rule of sacrificing animals for forgiveness of sins is no longer in force, but people have tended to substitute it with another act—self-effort in the way they govern their lives. They view the doing of good deeds, that is, being good people, as the way to God. Not that good behavior is to be ignored. The Bible is replete with instruction on ethical living. Practicing it is for everybody's welfare. But it doesn't meet God's standard for a saving relationship with him, a state that can only be obtained his way, not ours. And his way is that of grace.

Unfortunately, grace is predominately a foreign concept to people. That is because human society is built around getting things through self-effort. Working to attain a goal is ingrained in us from childhood, and I suspect that is true in most if not all cultures of the world. We learn that if we want success, we work at it, like studying hard to get good grades, or being diligent at the workplace in order to get a raise and promotion. We then carry it over erroneously to the spiritual and say, "It's what we *do* that reaps reward from God." It conjures up the idea that God helps those who help themselves.

No longer is that kind of thinking valid. The Bible clearly states that under the new covenant initiated through Christ, it is now God who does the work. What is left to us is to receive the benefit—the forgiveness of our sins and resulting gain of eternal life. It is cause for widespread jubilation. No wonder the angel announced the birth of Jesus to the shepherds by saying,

> I bring you good news of great joy . . . a Savior has been born to you; he is Christ the Lord. (Luke 2:10–11)

Why "good news of great joy?" Because the baby was to be a "Savior," or, "rescuer," meaning of course one who saves or rescues. And if he is to do that, it must mean that some people need rescuing. Not just a few, but everyone, including me, since the Bible states that "all have sinned" and as a consequence are separated from God (Rom. 3:23).

For restoration to take place, God demands a sacrifice. In Old Testament days, the sacrifice took the form of an animal offering, the blood of which God considered an atonement for sin (Lev. 17:11). In the New Testament, or new covenant, God specified another way—replacing the animal with a person, not just anyone, but his own Son. Scripture declares that the Father sent Jesus to earth to be sacrificed for the sins of the entire world (John 3:16). Christ took our misdeeds on himself to make us acceptable to the Father. In other words, he performed an act of substitution, which he did out of compassion for people. It was an act of love, an action of such magnitude that it defies full comprehension. Don't think it was easy just because God-man was doing it. Remember Jesus' agony in the garden of

Gethsemane just prior to his Crucifixion. Don't think that being pinned to a cross in itself was bothering him, as horrible and painful as that was. He was sweating blood in Gethsemane just before the cross because he, God-man, perfect in every way, without sin, was about to take on himself the sins of the entire world and consequently be forsaken by the Father in the process. That is why he uttered in his dying moments,

> My God, my God, why have you forsaken me? (Matt. 27:46)

Can you imagine? The Creator himself dying for his creation? The apostle John saluted Jesus for doing that.

> To him who loves us and has freed us from our sins by his blood. (Rev. 1:5)

The Bible defines it as "grace." It is God's graciousness to us . . . redeeming us from our lost state that separates us from God. It should cause us to cry out in thanksgiving and praise.

Let it sink in! Grace says that God made the sacrifice, not us. It was a single yet all inclusive one that brings us into harmony with him. Human effort in working at it (sacrificing) through good deeds or through rules and regulations is no longer valid. It is in fact an insult, a slap in the face to God, because it says: "I'll do it my way. I don't like yours."

Self-effort is a common philosophy in today's society. It was made so clear to me recently through a nationally televised show which discussed the question, "Do you need to be a Christian to go to heaven?" The program revealed mass confusion over the issue, as it included multiple input from the panel of "experts," the audience, and outside telephone callers who continually reverted to the idea of attaining heaven through good deeds.

If you were to take a poll on the subject of going to heaven, you would more than likely be told, as I have, of the need to be good. Typical answers are: "I hope I'll go to heaven, because I'm not a bad person;" or, "I try to help others;" or, "I try to be good;" or, "I'm a churchgoer." That mentality is also reflected in jokes in which St. Peter, standing at heaven's gate, queries people on their merits for entrance. Doing good deeds, the exact opposite of God's way of a free gift, is viewed as the ticket to heaven.

It is an incredible mix-up. The New Testament has been around for some 2000 years proclaiming salvation by grace. Yet humanity, as it seeks God's acceptance (if it chooses to do so at all), selects another route—self-effort. In contrast, Christianity loudly proclaims that it is God's effort that counts. The only effort involved for us is to accept it.

One further characteristic of "grace" helps us better appreciate God's work on our behalf. Embedded in the word is the connotation of a favor undeserved, often referred to as unmerited favor. That means we in no way deserve it, but God gives it to us anyway. In fact, the Bible declares God's graciousness by saying that he *lavishes* it on us. That is the way the apostle Paul described it to the Ephesians:

> In him we have redemption through his blood, the forgiveness of sins, in accordance with *the riches of God's grace that he lavished on us* with all wisdom and understanding. (emphasis mine) (Eph. 1:7–8)

It is an extravagant act, because God really ought to lambaste us for our sins. Instead, he just pours out his grace without holding back, which includes forgiveness for our foul-ups. That is why people often refer to the gospel as the Good News of Grace.

The idea of "good news" is a good way of looking at grace. It is inherent in the Greek word "gospel" (*euaggelion*), which signifies "good news." The apostle Paul defined the gospel as Christ's death, burial and resurrection . . . all for the purpose of restoring our relationship with God (1 Cor. 15:1–5). But this is only good news if we believe/receive it (John 1:12). After all, a gift is no good to anyone who doesn't accept it. Why would anyone want to tell God to get lost, that his gift of grace is not wanted? It is the greatest give-away on earth.

But grace doesn't stop with salvation. It goes beyond the promise of heaven as it gives us the ability to cast off stubborn, selfish habits we acquired before becoming Christians. It is certainly good news for those seeking escape from alcohol and drug abuse, sexual immorality, and other body and mind destroying acts. But it also gives joy to those needing deliverance from more commonly found practices of anger, hatred, lying, selfishness, and a host of other negative behaviors declared throughout Scripture as robbing us of peace and happiness God wants us to enjoy.

It is all tied to our initial act of belief in the Savior that sets us free from our old selves and gives us the resources to start a new life. Listen to what God says about it!

> Therefore, if anyone is in Christ, he is a new creation; the old has gone, the new has come! (2 Cor. 5:17)

There is power in Christ to start anew, no matter what be our need.

Law Versus the New Covenant

Here is where we can get ourselves into trouble. Well-meaning but confused Christians often go about defining certain behaviors they think must be a part of the newness of life in Christ. They do it by reinstating Old Testament Law and establishing rules and regulations from it to form a part of what they think is Christian living. We get insight into the mistake of making Christianity a rule-oriented religion by reviewing some happenings in early Christendom.

After Jesus' resurrection and ascension to heaven, the Christian faith spread rapidly. People recognized their spiritual need, and were convinced that Jesus was the way to God. We see recorded in Luke's writing entitled "Acts" that although Christ's message was first directed to Jews, it was later extended to Gentiles who vastly outnumbered Jews. That inclusion of non-Jews set the stage for an interesting event to come about.

The Bible tells us that Judaizers (Jews who tried to influence Gentile Christians to adopt Jewish customs and beliefs) began teaching Gentile believers to incorporate commandments of the Old Testament Law into their way of living (Acts 15) (Galatians). They wanted to put requirements on them, such as the rite of circumcision, that in effect would have diminished the full meaning of Christ's work on the Cross. They saw Christ's sacrifice as only a starting point for getting right with God rather than as a complete act of redemption.

The problem with the "starting point" idea is that the requirements added to it make Christianity a rule-keeping religion. Incorporated in it are mandates supposedly reflecting spiritual living but in essence detract from and even minimize the cross death of Christ. That is a serious error in that it chips away at God's grace. It says in essence that Christ's death is not sufficient in itself for uniting us with God, but that we must add to it by doing things.

It may be that some of these people were well-meaning Jews who found it difficult to completely substitute their beloved law with their new faith in Christ. But the apostles would have none of it. They knew that Christ through his death completed the way of salvation, and that it need not be added to in any way. The apostles understood that God had established a new covenant which, in contrast to the old, allowed a freedom from rules heretofore unknown under the decrees of the Old Testament.

The matter was settled in the Council of Jerusalem, a meeting of the apostles and church leaders. Peter got up and made a remarkable statement:

> Now then, why do you try to test God by putting on the necks of the disciples a yoke that neither we nor our fathers have been able to bear? No! We believe it is through the grace of our Lord Jesus that we are saved, just as they are. (Acts 15:10–11)

Here Peter was emphatic. He stood strong for grace, something absolutely different from the Law and its characteristics of subjugation and bondage (a "yoke"). He would have none of the foolishness of requiring the Jewish rite of circumcision as necessary for salvation, or for that matter, of applying any aspect of Old Testament Law to Christians (v. 5). Paul reminds us that Christ through death took care of all that.

> Having canceled the written code, with its regulations that was against us and that stood opposed to us; he took it away, nailing it to the cross. (Col. 2:14)

That means that just as Jesus was nailed to the cross, so was the Law. The cross death of Jesus provided a freedom from rules as a standard procedure for Christians to follow.

> It is for freedom that Christ has set us free. Stand firm then, and do not let yourselves be burdened again by a yoke of slavery. (Gal. 5:1)

Burdened? Yoke? Slavery? Paul, how dare you use such words! And on top of it the writer of Hebrews had the audacity to say that the Law is to be put aside "because it was weak and useless" in perfecting us according to God's standard. (Heb. 7:18). No, these men were not being facetious. Nor were they slamming the Old Testament as being void of worth. What they were doing was underscoring the vast difference between the old and new covenants in making us righteous in God's eyes. They were holding fast to grace teaching; that is, that the way we begin and continue a relationship with God is not by following rules but by accepting complete perfection through Jesus' sacrifice.

James stood up to second Peter's pronouncement about the inappropriateness of applying law teaching to Gentile Christians. The meeting ended with the apostles, the elders and the whole church in accord, communicating to the Gentile believers that they were not to mix living by rules with New Testament grace. Grace won out. The Bible tells us there was joy among the Gentiles upon hearing it (v. 31). And why wouldn't there be? Peter had just labeled Old Testament rules an unbearable "yoke." Those words rang clear for the Gentile Christians, who must have been hoping the Gospel of Christ would grant freedom from self-effort. And they were right. God's new covenant had come into effect. Its starting point was Jesus' death.[1] You may remember Jesus being at the last meal with his disciples before his arrest and crucifixion. He held up a cup of wine, saying,

> This is my blood of the covenant, which is poured out for many for the forgiveness of sins. (Matt. 26:28)

His blood (death) initiated the new covenant we can all enjoy. The idea of striving to gain God's approval was now substituted by Christ's work on the Cross. Good news! No more imposition of legalistic demands to bring us and keep us in good stead with our Creator. Let's rejoice in that fact, and then live by it.

A New Commandment

If we are not to follow a set of rules, such as those demanded of Old Testament Jews, how shall we govern our behavior? The grace of Christianity surely has to involve more than taking a gift from God and then living whatever way we want. That is hardly showing gratitude. The entire process is wrapped up in one single command spelled out by Jesus:

> A new command I give you. Love one another. As I have loved you, so you must love one another. By this all men will know that you are my disciples, if you love one another. (John 13:34–35)

Some people interpret that command as one to be tacked on to the hundreds (613, in fact) given to the nation of Israel in the Old Testament. To make matters worse, they misconstrue some of the other commands given by Jesus by failing to view them within their proper context.

How important context is! A case in point is the one in Matthew (7:1) that enjoins us not to judge others—a command widely but mistakenly cited to answer insinuations of inappropriate behavior. "Don't you correct me," they say. "The Bible says not to judge." They fail to view the context of Matthew 7, which has to do with people judging others when they themselves are guilty of the identical behavior. Furthermore, a major thrust of the entire New Testament is that we look out for one another's spiritual welfare . . . to do it gently, of course . . . but to accept it as a God-given responsibility.

Another of Jesus' statements, especially cited as justification for holding to a command-oriented Christianity, is that of obedience to his teaching. John records it in his gospel.

> If you obey my commands, you will remain in my love. (John 15:10)

That puts a high priority on obedience, it would seem. But it does nothing more than exemplify the danger of isolating biblical statements and pulling them out of context. Just two verses later, Jesus explains his previous declaration by saying,

> My command is this: Love each other as I have loved you. (v. 12)

In other words, he lumps all commands into one—love. He is defining his statement: "Obey my commands." The practice of love fulfills all his commands because it regulates life to the extent of combating all unwanted behavior.

John, in his first epistle, also addresses this phenomenon of love as the means of fulfilling obedience to commands. He begins by stating a seeming contradiction:

> We know that we have come to know him if we obey his commands. (1 John 2:3)

A misreading of that Scripture would be to declare that Christians must observe a host of rules to prove the genuineness of their faith, and that if they don't measure up they will get clobbered. That would be totally contradictory to the gospel of grace. We must read on to allow John to explain himself in the totality of his teaching. He quickly defines the meaning of "obey his commands," as he lumps all commands into one, just as Jesus did.

> And this is his command: to believe in the name of his son, Jesus Christ, and to love one another as he commanded us. (1 John 3:23)

Believing and *loving* are the key elements here. You may want to reread the passage to see how those words stand out. They unlock the door to understanding Christian behavior. That means that after accepting God's grace for salvation through Jesus, we operate in accord with our inner dictates of love. Elsewhere in the New Testament, love is explained as a product or fruit of the Holy Spirit who takes up residence in every believer (Gal. 5:22), which in essence means that if we listen to the Spirit, we will love. The extent of that love, of course, will show itself in accord with our willingness to follow the Spirit's bidding. But that is another matter which we will deal with later.

Faith in Christ followed by its enactment through love is the message Paul wanted to send when he said,

> The only thing that counts is *faith* expressing itself through *love*. (emphases mine) (Gal. 5:6)

In other words, sincere faith for salvation is followed by a love-centered life. Paul presented that truth, by the way, to the Galatian Christians who previously were on the right path but now were adding Old Testament rule keeping as an assist to their faith.

> You were running a good race. Who cut in on you and kept you from obeying the truth? That kind of persuasion does not come from the one who calls you. (Gal. 5:7–8)

How appropriate it was for him to preface that statement by saying: The only thing that counts is faith expressing itself through love (v. 6). In other words, love is a product of sincere faith, and can't become a reality without it.

That was Jesus' major message. It zeroed in on love, which tells us that everything we do is to reflect that moral principle. It takes care of negative behaviors that Jesus spoke of, such as hypocrisy, criticism, selfishness, unforgiveness, retaliation, and other non-loving acts, all of which are combated by following Jesus' instructions to love. Look at what he said in another passage:

> Love the Lord your God with all your heart and with all your soul and with all your mind. This is the first and greatest commandment. And the second is like it: Love your neighbor as yourself. (Matt. 22:37–39)

Mark's gospel attached a fourth prepositional phrase to those of "loving God with all your heart, and with all your soul, and with all your mind." Love the Lord "with all your strength," he added (Mark 12:30). The obvious meaning is to love God with one's whole being, with intensity. That love carries over to our dealings with people, or as Jesus stated it: our "neighbor."

In other words, belief in Christ the Savior leads us to practice love by serving others. So critical is love as the all encompassing ingredient of Christianity that it constituted Jesus' parting message to his disciples at that significant event we call the Last Supper, when they met prior to Jesus' arrest and crucifixion (John 13). He didn't want them to forget the absolute importance of loving one another. Aside from believing in him as Savior, they were to practice love. He then demonstrated in practical terms a means of carrying it out—serving one another. And he didn't pull any punches as to the inclusiveness of serving. He exemplified it vividly by the lowly act of washing their feet. What a show of humility! Can you imagine? God Omnipotent, the Creator of the Universe, stooping to wash the feet of those very beings he created. I suspect the disciples never forgot that object lesson. Nor should we!

Controlling Sin

I hope you see the futility of following rules as the way to please God. The Bible is clear in teaching that rule-governed behavior is useless for gaining salvation as well as for living the Christian life. It is contrary to grace. In its stead is God's declaration that we please our heavenly Father by operating out of belief (faith) followed by love, which is the identifying feature of true faith.

I recognize, however, that people may accept love in principle, that is to say, to acknowledge its moral basis as one of life's ideals, without giving it much concern in terms of application. To do so is really to look myopically at the word's meaning. The result may be our failure to take seriously the sins the New Testament charges us to avoid. Let it be perfectly understood that, although under grace, we are still sinful beings and obliged to keep our imperfect nature under control (Rom. 8:6,8). Scripture spells it out more forcefully by telling us to put to death all manner of evil thinking and doing (Col. 3:5–10).

We might think that certain behaviors such as pride, drunkenness, greed, envy, jealousy, and selfishness are one's own business. And since those behaviors don't seem to openly involve others, we might think they don't violate Jesus' command to love others. Oh yeah? They may appear on the surface to be the exclusive business of their perpetrators, but they indeed go beyond one's personal life, because they do affect others, albeit indirectly. Think about possible repercussions on people, for example, if we are self-centered. How do you suppose our families are affected if we are drunkards, or if we are selfish in the amount of time we spend with our spouses and children?

Sins are cited in the New Testament, however, that are directly related to the abuse of others. Look at their listing: malice, slander, gossiping, dishonesty, lying, theft, rudeness, anger, bitterness, hatred, retaliation, hypocrisy, disobedience to parents, dissension and divisiveness, sexual immorality and murder. If we are honest, we will admit that some of these sins crop up in every one of our lives at times.

Does that mean that since they are sins affecting others we don't know Christ, as the apostle John seems to say? Absolutely not! Again, we must heed the entire biblical context on grace. As believers in Christ we are recipients of God's goodness, which means our eternal destiny has already been sealed (Eph. 4:30). Resting in grace is a marvelous position to enjoy, since it doesn't charge sin, any sin, against us. I like Paul's quoting of David in this regard:

> Blessed are they whose transgressions are forgiven, whose sin are covered. Blessed is the man whose sin the Lord will never count against him. (Rom. 4:7–8)

David knew temporary forgiveness of his sins through animal sacrifice, but God revealed to him the coming blessing of *complete forgiveness*—sins that "never count against him." That included sins that he and we would commit even in the future.

But an all-encompassing forgiveness doesn't free us from taking steps to live uprightly. Paul wrote the Roman Christians that, although their sins were covered by grace, they lacked good sense if they thought they could behave however they wanted. He reasoned that through Christ they had been made new, so why would they want to go back to their old ways? (Rom. 6:1–2). John seconded it by saying,

> We know that anyone born of God does not continue to sin. (1 John 5:18)

As recipients of grace, we don't abuse that marvelous goodness of God; rather we complement it by putting a check on our behavior. Grace brings freedom, and freedom involves responsibility, which is really an act of gratitude on our part for God's gift of grace. That is what defines a true believer from one merely claiming Christianity without living it. John's epistle sets the record straight:

> No one who is born of God will continue to sin, because God's seed remains in him; he cannot go on sinning, because he has been born of God. This is how we know who the children of God are and who the children of the devil are: Anyone who does not do what is right is not a child of God; nor is anyone who does not love his brother. (1 John 3:9–10)

It all ties in nicely with Jesus' conversation with Nicodemus: "You must be born again," Jesus told him (John 3:7). The new spiritual birth he was talking about turns one's life around. You don't become a robot in God's hands, because God always allows you to operate under free will. But the new birth makes it possible for you to be a new person, as God implants his "seed" in you. And that verifies you as a true child of God (2 Cor. 5:17).

I like what M. Scott Peck says about taking care how we behave—our self-control. He quotes St. Augustine, *Dilige, et quod vis fac*, and translates the last four words to mean: "and what you want do." *Dilige* translates, of course, to "Be diligent," but Dr. Peck thinks St. Augustine may have had in mind two alternative meanings: "Love!" and "Love God!" In other words, if you are diligently loving God, your actions, no matter what they be, will be moral and pleasing to God.[2] The interpretation may come under question linguistically, but it complements the apostle Paul's teaching about freedom in Christ. As recipients of God's grace, we have an entirely different outlook on how we live.

Therein lies the beauty of Jesus' new commandment to love. We put a check on our behavior when we operate under the principle of love, because we know it affects God, us, and others.

Human Rules

Some people, in their zeal for godly living, distort the whole picture of faith and love by creating their own rules which they inflict on themselves and on others too. It is a rather subtle error because they obey rules, they think, out of love for God. They become so zealous about turning from sin that they start inventing ideas as to what sin is. And then they start inflicting those ideas on others. The scenario is reminiscent of the Jewish religious leaders of the first century. Jesus lambasted them for religious traditions they had concocted which had nothing to do with following God (Matt. 15:6–9).

Today we see people making an indirect association of a given behavior with some scriptural passage and then declaring the behavior as sinful. This is done by inventing requirements (most of them taking a negative tone forbidding certain kinds of conduct) they believe to represent spirituality. Those rules often involve such acts as smoking, drinking, movie-going, dancing, card playing, mode of dress, hair length, "improper" use of the Sabbath, and many more. They deal with externals. A lot of them are never even mentioned in the Bible. All of them if avoided might give a semblance of spirituality, but they really amount to a crippling legal system of human origin that contradicts the simplicity of God's new covenant of grace. Paul warned Christians about people who make their own legal requirements:

> Therefore do not let anyone judge you by what you eat or drink, or with regard to a religious festival, a New Moon celebration or a Sabbath day. (Col. 2:16)

Such were some of the rules mistakenly imposed by Jewish legalists in the first century. Paul told Christians to stand up to anyone trying to do that to them. Some of those Christians were undoubtedly Jews who all their lives had been under a tight legal system. Now they were set free by the new covenant of grace. They were not to forget it.

I wish someone would have told me that when I was a young Christian. I remember certain conditions imposed on me that made Christianity a rather grim way of life. Don't get me wrong; I rejoiced in my newfound faith. It gave me the peace of knowing that God promised me heaven, an assurance I lacked before believing in Christ as my Savior. But the kind of life I was told to live was frankly a burden. It was a drag. I know personally why Paul used the term *burden* in writing to the Galatians:

> Do not let yourself be burdened again by a yoke of slavery. (Gal. 5:1)

Yes, and he even likened it to being hitched up to a yoke—a form of slavery. Below are a few personal examples. They may cause you to reflect on people-made rules having a grip on your life.

Sabbath Keeping

Growing up on the shores of Lake Erie, I liked the fun of spending a Sunday afternoon on the sandy beaches of Presque Isle State Park in Erie, Pennsylvania. On a warm, sunny day, it was almost automatic for me to say to Mom and Dad—"Let's go to the peninsula." (That's what we called it back then, and I think people still do today.) But when I became a Christian, I was told that beaches and swimming on "the Lord's Day" were inappropriate for a follower of Christ. A human law based on the fourth of the Ten Commandments ("Remember the Sabbath day by keeping it holy") was being interpreted and imposed on me as a standard for Christian conduct. It was, as if to say, that Sunday activities were to consist of only serious and somber ones. You were not to have fun on the Sabbath.

Here are some other examples in support of my thesis: (1) Given two passes to the Pirates' Sunday afternoon baseball game, Howard invited Rick, his church buddy, to attend the event. Rick turned him down because "it's not the Christian thing to do on Sunday;" (2) Bob and Jane, new students at X Christian College, trotted off to the campus tennis court Sunday afternoon for some ball lobbing, only to find the gates locked and then being told by a passing security guard that "tennis was not allowed on the Lord's Day;" (3) Jimmy wanted to go fishing with his friends, but Mom objected, saying without explanation, "It's not something you do on Sundays;" and, (4) Billy wanted to apply for the paper route that had just opened up in his neighborhood, but his Dad said no. "But Dad," Jimmy pleaded, "it won't interfere with church. I can throw the papers at 6:00 AM, in plenty of time for Sunday school and church." Dad replied, "We don't work on Sundays."

I grew up with those kinds of restrictions. My joy killers, who happened to be fellow church members, wouldn't let go of the rigorous Old Testament command about Sabbath keeping. (Actually, that command was far more rigid than they imagined—it prohibited work of any sort on the Sabbath, including gathering wood for cooking or for whatever, and demanded the death sentence of the violators.) (Ex. 20:8; 31:15) (Num. 15:32–36). My fellow church members might be compared to the Pharisees of Jesus' time. Those first-century zealots of Judaism invented a host of regulations they thought explained the Law more fully. But Jesus condemned them, saying that their manmade traditions actually nullified God's Word (Matt. 15:6). In other words, we cancel God's intent by adding our own rules to Scripture, and thus establish our own legal code on how the Christian life is to be lived. There is nothing wrong with tradition, but when it interferes with Scripture, it must go. Those first-century Jewish leaders had actually created religious traditions beyond the Mosaic Law, and they imposed them on their fellow Jews. Look at the following account.

> The Pharisees and some of the teachers of the law who had come from Jerusalem gathered around Jesus and saw some of his disciples eating food with hands that were "unclean," that is unwashed (The Pharisees and all the Jews do not eat unless they give their hands a ceremonial washing, holding to the tradition of the elders. When they come from the marketplace they do not eat unless they wash. And they observe many other traditions, such as the washing of cups, pitchers and kettles.) So the Pharisees and teachers of the law asked Jesus, 'Why don't your disciples live according to the tradition of the elders instead of eating their food with unclean hands?' He replied, 'Isaiah was right when he prophesied about you hypocrites; as it is written: These people honor me

> with their lips, but their hearts are far from me. They worship me in vain; *their teachings are but rules taught by men.*' (emphasis mine) (Mark 7:1–7)

I hope that last phrase—*their teachings are but rules taught by men*—has registered with you. Jesus' message comes forth loud and clear: Be on guard against those who invent spiritually sounding laws that put you under bondage contrary to God's covenant of grace.

Dancing

Here is another example of the kind of foolishness I was told to submit to in my early years as a Christian. It had to do with the "sin" of dancing. I didn't dance myself; any attempts at it were such as though I was born with two left feet. I was an unmitigated disaster on the dance floor. Nevertheless, I contributed to others engaging in that activity through my role as a musician in a swing band. (I still remember with fondness the melodies of the big band era of the 1940s.) But "dancing is not Christian," I was told. "Christians are not to participate in activity allowing embrace between unmarried males and females." And what's more, if you were married you wouldn't want to be seen in the ballroom out of fear of influencing singles.

So I was compelled to quit the band. Far be it that I should contribute to others sinning. After all, even the preacher was voicing that opinion. But I had a feeling that somehow that rule imposed on me was not quite right.

When I share this story with younger people today, I get reactions of disbelief, together with sympathetic smiles. What's more, we look on dancing differently today. Christian couples from evangelical churches actually take lessons on ballroom dancing, the kind done in the 1940s. Is it okay for them to dance that way today? It wasn't back then.

What does that tell us of people's rules and their application from one era to another?

I recognize there may be individual differences in how Christians look at dancing. And certainly anyone with any sense would rule out body movements of a sexually inciting nature. The point is that we can cause a lot of harm by establishing a spiritual behavior for ourselves, and then hoisting it on others too. It is one of those areas on which the Bible is silent. We must leave it to one's liberty in Christ to decide on its appropriateness for his or her life. If we insist on our own petty reasoning about right and wrong, we can do a great deal of harm.

Movies

Another problem thrown at me in my early Christian life had to do with moviegoing. It represented yet another condemnation made by my church and even imposed by the Christian college I attended. With the latter, I had to sign a pledge stating that, were I granted admission, I would not go to movies. It wasn't just a question of selecting appropriate films to see; all movies were included..

Then came movie replays and other drama on television, and the college requirement had to be rescinded (really rephrased, to save face, I guess). I am sure you are beginning to see why I am so strong on grace and staunchly against its opposing legalism. People-made rules about appropriate Christian conduct obviously don't hold up from one era to another. That in itself ought to tell us something about our puny understanding of a Christian lifestyle when we condemn certain behaviors in the first place. Furthermore, trying to follow those rules often does harm by giving a false sense of spirituality.

Condemnation of movies of course couldn't be made on the basis of any of the Bible's commandments. But it was justified by citing the non-Christian behavior depicted in the films. Therefore it became a commandment, one held by my church back then. Today I occasionally watch the television replays of those movies of the '40s and '50s, and oh how innocent they are! (I must admit, however, how ridiculous the actors seem as they almost continually light up those white four-inch protrusions hanging limply from their lips, an action that comes across as quite silly and comical in light of society's general rejection of cigarettes today.)

I want to make it clear that it is not my intent to encourage moviegoing. I have seen recently produced films whose flagrant display of sex, violence and other unwholesome behaviors have turned me away in disgust. I also suspect that immersion in watching those behaviors wields a negative influence on us, just as Scripture says:

> Bad company corrupts good character. (1 Cor. 15:33)

My personal opinion is that society today, not only of the United States but of other countries as well, is in a state of moral decay, which I see caused largely by the unwholesome display of sex, violence, disobedience to parents, lack of discipline in the schools, and other havoc-creating behaviors depicted in movies, television, magazines and other media. If you see a lot of that stuff, you may succumb to it and believe it acceptable. But it is for you, the reader, to decide what constitutes a bad association. I have no right to make a law out of it and to impose it on others. I think, however, that there is truth in the adage that you eventually become what you associate with.

The point I want to make about legalistic demands is the toll they take on one's well-being. They were burdensome laws, made by people, and they robbed me of the joy of living according to God's design of liberty in Christ. Of course back then I knew nothing about Christian liberty. Instead I thought being a Christian meant a great deal of suffering and personal sacrifice, something akin to a monastic life of self-denial. At times I got so fed up with those harsh demands that I thought of walking away from the faith. Now that is serious.

Christians in Galatia got hung up on petty rules that interfered with grace, and it must have taken the zest out of them for the liberty afforded them in Christ. Paul had to ask what happened to all their joy (Gal. 4:15). I can picture them walking around with faces looking as if they were sucking lemons. Putting yourself under rules instead of the freedom of the new covenant will eventually do that to you. It is nothing less than a return to slavery. That is why Paul cried out saying,

> It is for freedom that Christ has set us free. Stand firm, then, and do not let yourselves be burdened again by a yoke of slavery. (Gal. 5:1)

Legalism has yet another danger—guilt. I suffered from it, and did it ever affect my joy. It is a wonder it didn't affect my sanity, since it seemed that every time I turned around a new prohibition was being imposed on me. Because of the indictment against movies in general, I even felt guilty later in life when I decided to see films of a religious bent, such as "The Robe" and "The Ten Commandments."

I remember approaching the theater's box office and looking about nervously out of fear of being seen by my legalistic friends who might happen to be passing by. That may sound funny to younger readers who never faced such prohibition. But what I am underscoring is the harm that comes about from a legal system concocted in the minds of "religious" people and imposed on others through their reading of certain scriptural passages (like 2 Corinthians 6:17–18) that urge us to avoid identifying with practices of unbelievers. It was supposed to represent separation from the world. And that psychological conditioning, if of lengthy duration, tends to keep its grip on you for a substantial period of time, just as it did with me, until I got insight into Paul's emphasis on Christian liberty.

But the saddest result of legalism is that, as we interpret the Christian life as a set of joyless, inhibiting rules, we may turn from devotion to Christ, just as I was tempted to do. It can happen out of bitterness toward those restrictions when you are made to believe that submission to them is a requisite for good standing with God. Such people come to a point of realizing that the offensive rules are nothing more than someone else's desire to assume control over them. The message of separation from the world keeps ringing in their ears. They feel deceived. They see Christianity negatively, and they no longer want association with it. What a terrible indictment on those who impose their legalism on others to the point of influencing the abandonment of Christianity.

But legalism not only affects Christians, but others too. How sad it is to see people rejecting the gospel message because of human concocted ideas defining Christian living. We Christians have an obligation to avoid mixing human-made rules with God's standards. It gives the world a negative perception of the Christian faith, and hardly induces one to investigate the true message of Christ.

Other Rules

Inventing rules on spirituality is not just something of the past; it erupts in various forms today. People seem to have a proclivity for creating codes of conduct to impose on others in the name of Christian living. Certain groups today propagate the same rules I had to bear as a young Christian: no movies, no card playing, no dancing, no smoking, no drinking, and no entertainment on Sunday. And they add others too, such as no television, no short hair on women, no long hair on men, no beards, no jewelry or makeup, and no absence from church on Sunday morning and evening, and maybe on Wednesday night too. The sad part of it is that some of these people not only view obedience to those rules as pleasing to God (some hold rejection of these rules as outright sin) but as necessary for salvation as well.

You may say that nobody follows such rules today. Well, I happen to know plenty of people who do. They talk about being under grace, but when pinned down, they show themselves under the control of human rules. The point I am trying to make is that we recognize the subtlety of setting up standards for Christian behavior based on faulty reading into a biblical passage. It is an ever present danger lurking in every American home and church. I will put you to the test on one such rule. See if it applies to you.

Do you raise your eyebrows if a fellow believer you are dining with drinks a glass of wine with his meal? You may say, sure! Doesn't the Bible say we shouldn't get drunk on wine? (Eph. 5:18) I agree wholeheartedly, that we shouldn't get *drunk* on it. But are we to assume that alcohol is always connected to excessive drinking because some people practice it? It seems important that we not carry our predetermined views into interpreting a given biblical passage. We tend to do that without realizing it, both favoring or opposing a given idea, in this case abstinence or consumption.

Evangelicals tend to regard alcohol suspiciously. By their dogmatism against it you would think that Jesus went to the wedding at Cana to change the wine into water. Total abstinence certainly has its roots in American Christianity. That tradition has a way of controlling our thinking on right and wrong. But we need to question whether abstinence from alcohol is a people-made rule or a biblical one. It seems important, given biblical instruction on liberty in Christ, that we protect that privilege while at the same time heed biblical admonition about misusing freedom to cause a brother to fall (Rom. 14:12). Who that brother might be is left for each of us to decide. Setting up a rule for all to obey is to impose a law of our own making, the kind Jesus condemned when he told the Pharisees that they nullified the Word of God because of their tradition (Matt. 15:6), and that their teachings were nothing more than rules of their own making (v. 9).

Some Christians are similarly guilty with rule making on abstinence. They are so concerned about the possibility of someone's weakness with alcohol that they condemn drinking it altogether. I would certainly not offer a glass of wine to an ex-alcoholic, or even drink in his presence. I recognize the temptation and danger for him. However, the Bible doesn't allow us to establish a rule on alcohol to apply to everyone. Some people do so, and in all fairness I understand their good intent. But we must all view it in the context of Christian liberty and avoid trying to make robots out of fellow believers regarding a human rule. Judging one's spirituality should never be suggested in this respect. A rule that prohibits alcoholic consumption exemplifies the subtleties of people-made rules to govern spiritual living. It is the kind of rule the Pharisees made for what they believed to be holy living. Jesus condemned the whole process.

We make yet other "Christian" laws—condemnation of contemporary Christian music, for example. We lump the excesses of some of its performers into condemnation of all new forms of musical expression. The hymns older folks grew up with, and the way they were rendered, are not the only ways of worshipping with music. Traditional melodies and rhythms may be the best for us, but not necessarily for others.

My son enjoys attending church with me when he visits from Houston. But he has a hard time enjoying the music of the traditional service. To make matters worse, my wife agrees with him. So I cart them both off to the contemporary service and I try to tolerate its music. The younger generation has a totally different musical taste. But I still haven't figured out where my 64-year old wife is coming from on it. I just keep smiling and letting her be her own person. I must admit, however, that she will also attend the traditional service with me, as she understands my preference for traditional hymns. That seems to be a good give-and-take arrangement.

Then there is the insistence on dress codes, especially for a worship service, stating that we ought to "dress up" out of respect for God. Well, I can understand somewhat where they are coming from on dress, having seen a lack of common sense in exhibiting the flesh, as per girls wearing shorts and halter tops or extremely tight sweaters to the worship service. We ought to be concerned about enhancing the environment for worship, not distracting from it. Women need to realize that their dress can be a problem for men. Champions of today's women's movements might say, "Tough! That's man's problem," which simply says to me that those women have more need for attitudinal change than on that pertaining to dress.

I will suggest one further rule evangelicals generally accept but which lacks biblical support. The practice is so widespread that I fear being judged a heretic to question it. We even see leading evangelists practicing it. I am referring to appeals for people to do such things as raise their hands to indicate a desire to accept Christ or to rededicate their flagging Christian lives. Or perhaps it is an appeal to "come forward" (to the front of the church) to get saved, where they may be asked to repeat a prayer. These manipulative devices are used for several reasons, such as, to give new believers a more vivid impression of their conversion, to allow for follow up with them, and to record the number of respondents.

The question looming before us is: How true to the Bible are these practices? Can you imagine Paul answering the Philippian jailor's inquiry about salvation by having him repeat a prayer? Or how about Peter asking the crowd at Pentecost to indicate acceptance of Christ as Messiah by raising their hands followed by coming forward? To insist on such procedures is to ask people who newly believe the gospel message to do something beyond faith. It might even suggest faith plus works. People-made rules! It is reminiscent of Paul's cry to the Galatians (1:6–9) that they had better rethink what they were doing by adding to the simplicity of the gospel. He called their additions "a different gospel," and he was "astonished" that they would even consider them. In fact, he condemned those who were party to making those additions.

A few years back I collected a number of gospel tracts and church literature on how to be saved. I totaled eleven different items that were stated as necessary for salvation. Some listed five, others four, and yet others three or two. None listed only one requisite—*believe*—maybe because the authors thought it would cause readers to claim belief without sincerity. Along with its requirement of offering a salvation prayer, one tract insisted that the prayer be said out loud. ("If you truly want the Lord to give you eternal life, tell Him out loud," it said.) As incredible as it sounds, another tract even listed membership in a local church as a requisite. I wonder which listing people should follow who want to become Christians. If they got hold of the wrong publication, where would that leave them?

Many people cite Romans 10:9–10 to defend the need to not only believe but to make a verbal confession or a public display of belief. It is important to recognize that this passage is the only one in the entire New Testament, as far as I know, that talks about a verbal confession, or I should say, what we construe to be a verbal confession. On that basis, I hesitate to declare such a requirement as doctrinal. In spite of the passage being an isolated instance on the subject, curiosity calls for some explanation.

I quote the Romans passage below followed by an explanation of it by Nick Kalivoda, a careful student and teacher of the Bible for some 60 years.

> That if you confess with your mouth, 'Jesus is Lord,' and believe in your heart that God raised him from the dead, you will be saved. For it is with your heart that you believe and are justified, and it is with your mouth that you confess and are saved. (Rom. 10:9–10)
>
> It is unfortunate that the translators did not place higher value on the context of Romans 10 to guide them in the translation of its prepositions from the Greek text. In the passages prior to Romans 10:9, Paul is comparing the righteousness of the law with the righteousness of faith. In regard to the latter he writes: But what does it say? "The word is near you, in your mouth and in your heart" (that is, the word of faith which we preach). (Romans 10:8 NKJV) The above quotation is from Deuteronomy 30:14. The statement employs the preposition "in" twice, but the same Greek word unfortunately is translated "with" in v. 9, leading Bible readers to con-

> clude that a public confession is mandated for salvation. The meaning of these passages might have been enhanced with consistent translation of this preposition, resulting in this suggested translation: That if you confess (the word) *in* your mouth that Jesus is Lord and believe *in* your heart that God raised him from the dead, you will be saved. (v. 9) The insertion of "the word "(above), which appears in the revised Greek text of Westcott and Hort, contributes to the intended meaning of the passage. The context suggests that those who heard the preaching of the word of faith and have that word in their mouths and in their hearts are being addressed. They are told to agree (confess) with the message that Jesus is Lord and was raised from the dead. The same reasoning applies to verse 10 where "in the heart belief is made to righteousness, and in the mouth confession (of the word) is made to salvation. The context of Deuteronomy 30:14 suggests that the children of Israel had God's word; it was in their mouths and in their hearts. (See Proverbs 3:3, Joshua 1:8) They needed no further revelation from heaven or from across the sea. Paul's concern was for his unsaved Jewish countrymen (v. 1) and he applies this passage to those in Rome who heard the gospel, but apparently failed to agree with it and believe it. In v. 10 he explains that belief would lead to righteousness (as v. 11 affirms) and that agreement (confession) with the word preached (v. 8) would result in salvation.[3]

The explanation is long but necessary for dispelling the idea of some kind of public demonstration of faith, such as "going forward" or saying a prayer. To be sure, those traditions are followed with the utmost sincerity. However, they are rules people have devised which contradict the Bible's declaration of salvation through faith alone. They complicate the simplicity of the gospel and chip away at God's gift of grace.

Our Challenge

The foregoing discussion in large measure is oriented around *knowledge* of God's declaration on grace. It is an important first step in understanding what is and what is not God's intent under his new covenant. That helps us avoid error about how we are saved. It also steers us away from thinking we have to apply the commands of the Mosaic Law to remain in good stead with God. It likewise causes us to understand the futility of following spiritually sounding rules invented by yourself, and maybe by others too, with no solid scriptural basis.

But then comes *application.* The Bible appeals to us to live by grace. To start with, that means we allow his grace to affect our lives to the extent that we receive God's acceptance without trying to help him out. Look at what the Bible says:

> Are you so foolish? After beginning with the Spirit, are you now trying to attain your goal through human effort? (Gal. 3:3)

We don't have to work at pleasing God. Rather, we come to grips with his grace that shouts out through his loud speaker system: **Christ lives in you!** (Gal. 2:20). It is incumbent on us to accept that fact! Jesus thinks so highly of us that he put himself in our bodies to inspire a walk in tandem with him. But we must not get confused. It is *he* who is going to perform. *Our* performance efforts are not only worthless but also harmful, because we will invariably fail at times, which will cause us to feel badly and want to give up. We turn it over to him to live through us just as he lives in us. In case we can't see it, that spells d e p e n d e n c y.

Having done that, we will be able to say, "Now we understand grace. It sets us free from ourselves". There is liberty in grace. Slavery to self-effort is out. Then we can really echo Paul's words:

> You, my brothers, were called to be free. (Gal. 5:13)

That in itself is much cause for rejoicing. But there is more to grasp. The next chapter, "Growing in Grace," will help us discover some of the means to enjoy the Christ life even further. It will be the *application* of grace to situations we encounter daily, which will give us greater appreciation of our God, who operates out of an indescribable love and concern for our well-being. That will make the Christian life even more meaningful, indeed one of spiritual health and resulting joy.

CHAPTER 2

Growing in Grace: The Dynamics of Christian Living

"And God is able to make all grace abound to you, so that in all things at all times, having all that you need, you will abound in every good work."

2 Corinthians 9:8

What does it mean to walk with God in grace? It goes beyond our previous discussion of accepting grace for salvation, and even acknowledging freedom from rules people may invent for "holy living." It takes us one step further—freedom from the tyranny of self and all that it encumbers. To grow in grace is to learn to rest in God rather than in our own designs. It is in effect a spectacular freedom God provides for each of his children. It is a part of the dynamics of Christian living.

I have not completely experienced this state of affairs. I am still learning. And that learning comes from my past mistakes which are often the best teacher. As a result, I am escaping a series of negative influences, some of which may be yours too.

Freedom from Guilt

I suppose we all look back on our lives at one time or another and feel guilty about some behavior. Unquestionably it is Satan's tool. He has lost the main battle when we put our faith in Christ for salvation. What is left for him is to try to destroy our ensuing Christian walk through subtle ways like memory of our past sins. Sin is a part of the natural man that God says carries over from Adam's disobedience (Rom. 5:12). Even the apostle Paul, although acknowledging forgiveness, still had to battle humanity's sinful nature. He admitted:

> I have a desire to do what is good, but I cannot carry it out. (Rom. 7:18)

He then proceeded to tell of God's gracious provision of freedom from condemnation (8:1). And believe me, he had reason to rejoice in that fact. We will get to that in a moment.

Many of us have a habit of delving into our negative pasts for self-condemnation. It does nothing more than play into Satan's hands to create guilt complexes and even to destroy the desire to pursue Christ-centered living. Satan whispers in our ears that we might as well forget this "glorified idea" about following Jesus. That is because he is what Jesus described as "a liar and the father of lies" (John 8:44). He revels in trying to confuse us. He glories in seeing us suffer. The tragedy of it is that we often concede to him, which we need not do, since God has made provision for our escape.

There has been nothing more evident in my feelings of guilt as I remember my early married life. I was an unmitigated disaster through self-centeredness as I failed to be a conscientious partner with my wife in the home. Kay was overwhelmed with the jobs of keeping the house clean, washing, ironing, marketing, cooking, and the like, to say nothing of the tremendous responsibility of caring for our five little ones. Why as a Christian husband couldn't I see what I was doing? Oh I saw it all right, but I justified my distancing by focusing on another aspect of what I thought was helping—developing my career so as to be a good financial provider. First it was getting the Master's degree, then the Doctorate, followed by burying myself in research to publish—a necessary requirement for a university professor to attain promotion in rank, increase in salary, and professional visibility.

There is nothing wrong with working hard to accomplish a goal. I thank God for the work ethic instilled in me by my parents during my youth. (I have always said I have more persistence than brains.) But going about it myopically without paying attention to how it affects others is when I run down the wrong path. How many people have been hoodwinked into thinking this way. Satan laughs. He sees the wife hurting. He loves it. Later he places on me a guilt trip as to my selfishness. I hurt. He loves it.

No excuse is acceptable for the foolishness of those younger days. Were I able to relive them I would of course do differently. But I can't go back in time. And the Lord took my wonderful, giving wife to her heavenly home before I had a chance to make things right. Now Satan would have me wallow in memories of self-centeredness. Why? He knows it makes me feel guilty, and he revels in doing that. You might say, "Good, you deserve it!" That is precisely Satan's message. It is one example of how the Devil works against me. There are hundreds of other ways too, of course. So what do I do about it? My hope lies in listening to what God says. His ways are different from those of my adversary.

God yearns for a relationship with me in which I increasingly recognize his available grace. The absolute first step in that process is to acknowledge *complete* forgiveness in Christ. When Jesus died he paid for *all* our sins, past, present and future. Because of his complete and perfect sacrifice he is described by the writer of Hebrews as a unique priest. Indeed, he is declared priest of God's new covenant.

> Day after day every priest stands and performs his religious duties; again and again he offers the same sacrifices, which can never take away sins. But when this priest had offered for all time one sacrifice for sins, he sat down at the right hand of God. (Heb. 10:11–12)

It was a complete and final act—Christ "offered for all time one sacrifice for sins." Then "he sat down at the right hand of God." There was no more work to do on his part. It was finished, just as he had proclaimed on the cross with his final breath. The writer continued saying that by Christ's sacrifice,

> He has made perfect forever those who are being made holy. (v. 14)

That is what makes the gospel so wonderful. Its meaning translated from the Greek is "good news." I have mentioned earlier that good news means freedom from the bondage of Old Testament laws as well as from "spiritual" rules made by people beginning with the first century and continuing to modern times. But good news also means that God has made us "perfect forever" through our faith in Christ the Savior. Of course we are not perfect in the sense that we can do nothing wrong. We still have our sinful nature carried over from Adam. But in God's eyes we are perfect, because we have chosen to believe in Christ for forgiveness of our sins. Our shortcomings are not charged against us. They in no way affect our eternal destiny. Neither do they affect God's love toward us as we go about our daily pursuits. That is the beauty of God's grace, enacted in a very special way through the death of Jesus Christ.

To allow ourselves to wallow in our shortcomings is to fail to acknowledge God's benevolent attitude toward our poor behavior. *He will not remember it* (Heb. 12:4). Somehow we have trouble coming to grips with that fact. We may do okay forgetting our sins prior to salvation, but we often find it hard to dispel guilt over sinning afterwards, especially when it hurts someone we love. Here is where grace shines through. God is always gracious even though we don't deserve it.

Let's face it. Although Christians, we still sin, we continue to do dumb things. It is a part of the natural man that carries over from Adam's disobedience. Even the apostle Paul, that strong defender of the faith, whom we esteem as perhaps the ultimate in spirituality, confessed his inability to live without sin. He knew that although he was forgiven through faith in Christ, he still had to battle humanity's sinful nature. That is why he declared,

> I know that nothing good lives in me, that is, in my sinful nature. For I have the desire to do what is good, but I cannot carry it out . . . What a wretched man I am! Who will rescue me from this body of death? (Rom. 7:18, 24)

His answer?

> Thanks be to God—through Jesus Christ our Lord. (v. 25)

In other words, he knew that through faith in Jesus he had God's complete forgiveness of his shortcomings, including any sins that may have continued to nag him. He proceeds to tell us of the gracious provision given through God's grace:

> Therefore, there is now no condemnation for those who are in Christ Jesus. (Rom. 8:1)

Do we understand what that means? No condemnation! Our Lord holds nothing against us. He may discipline us from time to time, but that is something different. It is not to get even, but rather to teach us what we would not learn any other way. He may want us to *stop* doing something. Or maybe it is something he wants us to *start* doing. He is our Father, and he disciplines us just as physical parents do with their children. He does it for our good (Heb. 12:5–11). But he holds no sin against us! All sins—past, present and future—are blotted out by Christ's blood on the Cross. It all has to do with that wonderful word "grace."

We are not condemned! Good news! But for many that notion is merely academic. We need to make it experiential. We read in the Scripture that says God maintains a totally forgiving attitude toward us. So how do we deal with past failures? How do we stop feeling guilty? How do we apply freedom from condemnation to the reality of life?

The Bible gives us practical advice. It counsels us to forget what is behind and to press on (Phil. 3:13–14). In other words, we concentrate on the future, not on the past! It is part of growing up in his grace. God inspired Paul to write:

> All of us who are mature should take such a view of things. (v. 15)

I imagine that as Paul wrote those words he may have been thinking of his own life. He not only experienced problems of sin as a Christian (Romans 7), but he undoubtedly had great sorrow over his life as a Jewish zealot before his dramatic conversion experience on the Damascus road. He committed horrible crimes—arresting and incarcerating Jewish Christians, and even contributing to their murder (Acts 26:9–11). We also have the account of his consenting to the fatal stoning of Stephen (Acts 8:1–3). He actually stood there giving approval to the death of that saint. He justified it all by reasoning that it was for the ultimate good of Judaism.

In his zeal to serve God, he was willing to kill those who differed with him. Just wipe them out. Nobody deserves to live if they transgress Judaism, was his judgment. All in the name of God. This believe-or-be-killed philosophy has been with us throughout the ages, as seen even today in the actions of Muslim terrorists.

I suppose if a Muslim terrorist converted to Christ, he might have grave feelings of guilt over the people he had murdered. Paul, in his zeal for Judaism, was no different. God teaches us through Paul's writings about guilt over past behavior. In essence he is saying, "Forget it! You made mistakes. Now put them behind you and live for Christ!"

That is great news for the brand-new Christian, because God has wiped away his sins, no matter how abominable they may have been. The same applies to those who commit sins after coming to Christ for salvation, or at least who do stupid things like I did with Kay. How does it apply? In the same way as with the new convert. Complete forgiveness! Of course we don't accept this good news flippantly, as if to fail to recognize the gravity of sinful ways. But we refuse to let the memory of sin destroy us. God has forgiven us. He doesn't hold our sins against us. Neither should we. That is one of the ways we live in God's grace. It is freedom from guilt. Satan can't stand seeing us do that.

I cite one further example to wrap up this section—that of Peter. If anyone had reason to feel guilty, it was Peter. He denied his Lord. Do you remember? Facing three accusations of being one of Jesus' followers,

> He began to call down curses on himself and he swore to them, 'I don't know the man!' Immediately a rooster crowed. Then Peter remembered the word Jesus had spoken: 'Before the rooster crows, you will disown me three times.' And he went outside and wept bitterly. (Matt. 26:74–75)

This was the man who accompanied Christ for three years. He had seen Jesus' miracles. He himself had performed spectacular events in the power of Christ's name (Matt. 10). He had witnessed all kinds of wonderful things happening to people through the power of God. In fact, he was the preacher on the day of Pentecost when Christ's words were fulfilled:

> But you will receive power when the Holy Spirit comes on you; and you will be my witnesses in Jerusalem, and in all Judea and Samaria, and to the ends of the earth. (Acts 1:8)

How did the Holy Spirit show himself? All the disciples began speaking in different languages to the foreign visitors in Jerusalem. Those foreigners marveled because they were hearing the wonders of God in their own languages.

Being personally involved in God's miracles, Peter would have had to be a real dumbbell not to be convinced that Jesus was the Son of God. But when the chips were down, when his own life was in danger, he denied his Lord.

It was a deadly moment for Peter, but probably not the only memory assailing him. He was human, just as we are, which means he continued to commit blunders. At that moment in denying his Lord he must have thought of himself as one big, stupid, ungrateful fisherman.

We all make mistakes, some big, some small, over which we grieve. But like Paul, Peter knew he had to put those memories behind him. He was not to hold on to them forever. He was not to let them destroy him. God had things for him to do. He knew that God was not holding his past against him. We are not to forget, Peter reminds us, that we are forgiven of all sins (2 Peter 1:9). Are you holding on to the memory of negative behavior in your life? God wants you to put the ugly past behind you. He wants you to experience the joy of living in the present in his grace. Yes, God has things for you to do too, just as he did with Peter, Paul and hundreds of other New Testament saints. What a beautiful picture!—you and Jesus, walking hand in hand.

But let's face the reality of the process. We are not to kid ourselves. Memories linger. They are not automatically destroyed through the act of confession, and Satan would have us dwell on them because he knows their destructive nature. On the other hand, we conquer those memories by claiming forgiveness and victory in Jesus—

> Forgetting what is behind and straining toward what is ahead. I press on. (Phil. 3:13–14)

Yes, we are realistic about recognizing our sins. But we don't let them conquer us. We press on, and God makes provision for our well-being. Let's always remember that through his grace—his gift to us—we have complete forgiveness!

Freedom from Self

A problem arises with forgetting the past. It is trying to do it in our own strength. Sure, resolve is involved. But if you are trying to do it by yourself, you won't like the results. That is because sometimes you will have success in blotting out unwelcome failures, but at other times you will fail. When the latter happens, guess what? Guilt intensified. That can drive you mad, because you are telling yourself that you are weak, wicked, and worthless—three bad w's. "Look at all the rotten things I've done," you say. "I've hurt so many people. I'm just not worth anything." Oh yes you are! In God's eyes you are special (and as a brother or sister in Christ you are special to me too; we are family). You are God's child, and you are loved. He wouldn't have implanted his Spirit in you—a mark of his acceptance—if he didn't esteem you highly.

The problem may be that you are forgetting God as your source of power. It is God, not you, who will put the past behind you. So how do you get that power? You already have it. You just may not have been utilizing it. If you haven't yet done so, tell God you realize that your own source of strength doesn't work. From now on you are leaning on Jesus . . . to let him work through you. And that applies not only to forgetting the past, but to conquering whatever negatives you may be presently experiencing.

Freedom from Anxiety and Fear

Let's look at another one of those negatives from which God through grace has set us free—anxiety. When allowed to go its own way, it causes fear. Anxiety and fear are really in opposition to grace. Who doesn't fall into this state from time to time? We know that Scripture admonishes against it:

> Do not be anxious about anything, but in everything, by prayer and petition, with thanksgiving, present your requests to God. (Phil. 4:6)

We worry anyway. We seem to have an automatic reflex toward it when things go wrong. Yet we know it does no good. In fact, it is harmful because of the toll it takes on us physically. Medical doctors warn us of the effects of worry on the circulation, the heart, the digestive system, and the entire nervous system. People actually die from worry.

Although my intent in this book is to discuss spiritual health, there is no question that following God's ways also brings physical benefits. That is one of the extra blessings we get as we heed his voice.

Our Creator knows what contributes to the malfunction of the human body. Why wouldn't he? He made us. What is his remedy to dispel worrying? We see part of it in his instruction to pray with thanksgiving. You may say, "I've tried praying, and it doesn't work." You are right it doesn't work, if you are praying *without* thanksgiving. You are overlooking a crucial component of prayer. When we have an attitude of thankfulness we appropriate God's grace to free ourselves from worry, no matter how bad the situation. That is what is meant in the rest of the Philippians passage:

> And the peace of God, which transcends all understanding, will guard your hearts and your minds in Christ Jesus. (Phil. 4:7)

Peace? It comes with trust. Let's get it in the right order. God honors trust by giving us peace. I don't know how he does it, but I know it happens. It is all a part of his grace. Paul, Peter, [illegible], James, and John all connected peace with grace as they greeted the brethren at the beginning of their epistles. Peter, for example, said,

> Grace and peace be yours in abundance. (1 Peter 1:2)

He not only uses the two words "grace" and "peace" together, but he emphasizes that they be ours "in abundance." How many times have you read that passage without thinking about the meaning of abundance? I am asking that question because I have read the passage hundreds of times without giving it much thought. Could Peter mean that we are not to fool around with the concepts of grace and peace by applying them superficially? And could he be using "peace" because he knew we would have it only in proportion to our acceptance of grace? Yes, I think he is saying that peace is an outcome of allowing God's grace to flow freely through us. We get it when we decide to come to grips with receiving grace. It is the same as with salvation. We get it only if we receive it. God offers peace. But it will not become a reality in our lives until we receive it.

The hard part is to accept peace in unwelcome situations. We don't like to have to bear them, nor do we like how they sometimes turn out in the end. But the verse seems to imply that even though God may not respond to our petitions in accord with our desires, we accept his response out of recognition that it is what he deems best.

We tend to have trouble with that kind of reasoning. To have to suffer through a painful situation is frustrating and even anger-inciting. But God doesn't hold our flawed responses against us. He is understanding; he knows our make-up. Look how he sacrificed by coming to earth to connect with us. The Bible clearly states that God through Jesus took on human form to share in our humanity. He did that in order to empathize with us (Heb. 4:15). The same passage tells us he sympathizes with our weaknesses. Thank God! But he doesn't answer our dilemma in any set way. He responds by granting our request immediately, or at a future time, or by not answering at all. Does the latter bother you?

Allow me to explain. An immediate healing of cancer, for example, brings great joy. Likewise, a more mundane experience of finding employment, be it a delayed response, is received happily. Suffering that leads to death, as in martyrdom, however, is hard to take. Christians are not exempt from it. Let's look for a moment at martyrdom to steer us toward responding to a situation of suffering. The Bible tells us that

> A time is coming when anyone who kills you will think he is offering a service to God. (John 16:2)

Indeed, the New Testament records martyrdom to be precisely what happened to John the Baptist and Stephen. And history tells us that other of Christ's early followers gave their lives for the faith in Roman coliseums, through crucifixion, burning at the stake, or in other ways devised by people's evil imaginations. Those who have died for Christ throughout the centuries are probably beyond count. Martyrdom even continues happening to many throughout the world today. Christians are having their lives taken because of their faith.

So Scripture foretells suffering and death of Christians at the hands of sinners. But unless we are among the few whose family members or friends have experienced such persecution, it doesn't really register with us. What does bother us is when we ourselves undergo a disastrous experience, as a life-threatening disease, for example, which God chooses not to heal. We would accept martyrdom (at least we think we would, since for most of us in the United States it is not within the purview of reality), but a death sentence at the hand of illness is inconsistent with a faithful God, we reason.

How do we resolve this dilemma? We have looked at the Philippians passage for what it says, but we may not have understood what it doesn't say. It contains no promise that God will fulfill a request, as small as it may be, as we think he should. Neither does it promise to fulfill our wishes as through something big, such as healing of a fatal disease. The passage does promise an inner peace when we make our request with thanksgiving.

I suggested earlier that a part of God's remedy lies in the Philippians 4:6 passage that speaks of maintaining an attitude of thanksgiving. Well, what is the other part? It is in the next verse that does not talk about something we must do but rather what God does. What is that? Peace! He makes it available to us.

> And the peace of God, which transcends all understanding, will guard your hearts and your minds in Christ Jesus. (Phil. 4:7)

God provides peace; we benefit by it in proportion to how we receive it.

Paul also speaks of peace as he tells the Philippians to trust God, which inevitably shows itself in the way we approach God in prayer. It is a matter of learning how to pray—bringing our requests to God *with thanksgiving*. It is an act of dependence on him without conditions or predetermined answers, even in the most ugly of circumstances.

I suspect that is what Paul and Silas were doing when thrown into prison. They didn't say, "we can get out of here in such-and-such a way, so let's ask God to help us do it." In no way were they going to dictate to God on how to free them. They weren't even about to ask God to set them free at all. Instead, what did they do? They sang hymns (Acts 16:25), in all likelihood ones of praise and thanksgiving, to rise above their circumstances. They didn't like being in jail. Who does? Especially in a Roman one, which I suspect was harsh and painful. Paul and Silas simply put their predicament in God's hands and were willing to live with the outcome. That was Paul's way, and it was likely passed on to Silas. But beyond giving them the power to accept imprisonment, God added an extra benefit—an earthquake that unlocked the prison doors. And on top of that, the jailer and his whole family became Christians. I can hear Paul and Silas telling each other, "It was worth it, wasn't it?"

Do you remember the words of the Philippians passage about praying with thanksgiving? That means we come before the Father with an attitude of resignation to his will, not insisting on our desires. It is trust, pure and simple. It is saying, "I trust you no matter the outcome." We may not completely understand the result at the time, or even until we unite with the Lord in heaven. But when we trust, we in effect acknowledge God's sovereignty and our acceptance of his will. God then does his part—he whispers his love toward us and grants us peace with which only believers can identify. He gives it to the martyrs, to the sufferers of cancer, to those told they have only six months to live, as well as to those with lesser difficulties. The world can't understand it, because it doesn't know the Savior and therefore is without the indwelling Holy Spirit to help them make sense of it all. Scripture describes it as a peace that transcends all understanding (Phil. 4:7).

That is the kind of peace Jesus referred to when he said,

> Peace I leave with you; my peace I give you. I do not give to you as the world gives. Do not let your hearts be troubled and do not be afraid. (John 14:27)

It is a promise of God. It is freedom from anxiety and fear. Even the Old Testament proclaims it:

> I will fear no evil, for you are with me. (Ps. 23:4)

And also:

> He will have no fear of bad news; his heart is steadfast, trusting in the Lord. His heart is secure, he will have no fear. (Ps. 112:7–8)

We will have this freedom from anxiety and fear when we come to grips with approaching God in all things with thanksgiving. We have it because of God's grace, which makes the fourth chapter of Hebrews a reality:

> Let us then approach the throne of *grace* with confidence, so that we may receive mercy and find *grace* to help us in our time of need. (emphases mine) (Heb. 4:16)

There is mercy in God's grace. It is not necessarily given for fulfilling our wishes for some spectacular act such as healing. It may well be in the form of such a miracle, but then it may not. Instead it may be an overwhelming inner peace, one that binds us closer to our Lord as we increasingly recognize his sovereignty, which includes acceptance of his knowing what is best for us. We see that involved in approaching the throne of grace with confidence. It says, God is in control! It doesn't say, Ask me whatever you want. Just press the magic button. I may not understand the rationale behind his decision making, but that doesn't affect the fact that he is working with superior knowledge.

I am compelled to give you one further idea about praying with an attitude of thanksgiving. Although I am learning to submit my prayer requests with a thankful heart, I often lose sight of that important principle as I go about the activities of the day. In other words, I find myself giving thanks during my secluded prayer time, but I often fail to do so throughout my daily activities. That may be why Paul admonished:

> Be joyful always; pray continually; give thanks in all circumstances, for this is God's will for you in Christ Jesus. (1 Thess. 5:16)

The passage speaks of actions I must initiate:

1. *Be joyful always.* That represents a conscious effort on my part to maintain a happy, positive attitude. Reminding myself of God's expression of grace and love in so many different circumstances in my life instigates an attitude of joy. What is the alternative? Walking about as if I were sucking lemons. That does no good for me nor for those with whom I come in contact. Instead, I appropriate God's joy that he extends to all who would have it.
2. *Pray continually*. Giving God thanks is not restricted to formal prayer time in my study. I practice it spontaneously throughout the day, maybe just a minute here or a few seconds there, as I see God's grace in operation.
3. *Give thanks in all circumstances.* That means, in everything—good and bad alike. Granted, it is harder to do in unwelcome circumstances, but it is effective in helping us override them. That includes giving thanks in even a string of hurts. I have to catch myself in that regard; I may be victorious in giving thanks over one grievous situation, but when another one comes about on top of it, I tend to tell God, "Why this second hurt? Isn't one enough?" In the back of my mind I am thinking that God caused it all. I must remember to give thanks in all

> circumstances, even though they are hurtful ones that pile on top of each other. The alternative is to moan and groan about them, to feel sorry for myself, and worse, to listen to Satan's message that God doesn't care. Depression and even anger set in.

The Thessalonians passage ends with, "this is God's will for you." Why do you suppose it says that? God is always interested in our well-being, so he gives us a prescription for good spiritual health. It takes us off the hook for responsibility of life's happenings (we relinquish them to God), and it paves the way for an attitude of joy. But that joy is something *we* have input into also; *we* must act upon it with a positive attitude. It is putting faith into practice, faith in God's grace. It is a lesson that Paul learned.

> I can do everything through him [Christ] who gives me strength. (Phil. 4:13)

God doesn't want us to be beset by worries or anxieties, but to override them. A joyful stance will give God glory in unimaginable ways. We will not have to see the outcome, but it will be there as it affects people all around us.

Glen, a friend and former faculty colleague, whose fall into a cavern several years ago resulted in his partial paralysis, is an example to me about joy in all circumstances. Wheelchair bound, nevertheless maintaining a positive attitude, he radiates joy in the Lord, which causes me to forget my puny problems. His attitude is a ministry in itself. It is a powerful example of giving thanks in all circumstances.

"Be joyful always," the Scripture declares. We should strive to make that our attitude. It will not only lift our spirits, but it will also affect those with whom we come in contact. Happiness is contagious. It is a ministry without words.

I am reminded of the story of the monk who decided to go to town to preach. He greeted people cheerfully who passed by, he joined with children in their play in the street, he stopped to pet a dog, and with peace and joy he contemplated a wild flower as people curiously looked on. On the road back to the monastery, his accompanying friend said, "I thought you were going to town to preach?" "I did," responded the monk.

The apostle Paul gives us one final challenge about our attitude in approaching God with thanksgiving (and confidence) as a prelude to internal peace. He tells us bluntly to put it into practice. Peace is one of God's gifts of grace, a fruit of the Spirit (Gal. 5:22). It is a blessing for us to appropriate whatever be the circumstances. It is there for us, but we must respond to it. It will be to our joy which, by the way, is another fruit of the Spirit.

The apostle Peter picked up on this theme of inner peace by saying,

> Cast all your anxiety on him because he cares for you. (I Peter 5:7)

Do you think doing that doesn't bring peace? Let me tell you of my personal experience with this concept.

I took early retirement from the University of Georgia to care for my late wife Kay who was in the beginning stages of a dreaded terminal disease. Shortly thereafter, I received a phone call from the President's Office of a Pennsylvania college asking if I would consider coming out of retirement to accept a teaching post there. They knew I was a Christian who would complement the college's spiritual emphases. I was honored by the request, but I dismissed it outright in view of Kay's illness.

A few weeks later, they called again inviting me to the campus "to take a firsthand look at the school's spiritual orientation." "Whoa!" I said to myself. Then a string of thoughts flooded my mind. "Is there something behind this that I'm failing to recognize? First they call me out of the blue to offer me a teaching post, and then they call again to see if I would change my mind. Why would they do that, calling twice? I thought I had made it clear I had caregiver responsibilities." But I couldn't help but wonder if God was behind this second call. Wanting to be open to his direction, I prayed, discussed it with Kay, and then followed through on an inner instinct to take the trip. Sometimes we do such things just to explore a feeling we have within us—a sensation that just might be from God.

Some degree of anxiety probably always exists in such situations. For Kay and me, this was one of inquiry to determine if God wanted us in Pennsylvania. I didn't need a job. I had taken retirement to be Kay's caregiver. But God had other plans.

Three days on the campus caused me to sense God's involvement in this new venture. Students and professors alike were open to spiritual fellowship, and the administration prized the way I related my faith to academics. Furthermore, Kay's mother and sister lived 70 miles down the road, facilitating frequent visits. But there was one thing that troubled me.

Sleepless in bed the night before returning home, I called out to God saying, "What a wonderful place to put my academic skills to work for you, but since there is no facility to care for Kay, how can I accept this job?" I then proceeded to tell the Lord that I trusted him for the outcome, whatever it would be. No demands. No suggestions. Just trust.

And if he provided no solution, I would return contented to Georgia. The response? An overwhelming feeling of peace such as I had never experienced. It was as if God were telling me to go to sleep and quit worrying. Through words reminiscent of 1 Peter 5:7 came the heavy impression of God saying, "I care. Trust me!" There were no promises. Just a feeling that I should resign myself to his will. That resulted in the peace that Paul spoke of to the Philippians. It was a calm that only God could give.

I awakened the next morning to the rustling about of the nurse (my room was in the college infirmary; I still smile over those "guest" quarters). During our coffee conversation I related my predicament. She knew of an excellent nursing/personal care home nearby, but it was only for permanent residents. Nevertheless, she suggested I inquire there, that maybe they would know of a way to meet my needs. I called immediately and was asked to discuss the problem with them face to face. The outcome? I still remember the exact words: "We've never taken in a day care patient, but something tells us we're supposed to step in here. Yes, doctor, if you're willing to be a pioneer, we'll be glad to take care of your wife." I couldn't believe what I was hearing, and in the last hours of my campus stay at that. I walked out of that facility, lifted my eyes to the heavens, and said, "Lord., how great you are." I cried.

Returning home, I told Kay of my experiences, but minus the nursing home incident for fear of influencing her decision. Her response? "Let's go!"

That is not the end of the story. Attending an all-college faculty meeting after my first month on campus, I decided to announce the formation of a faculty and spouse sharing group in my home for any who might be interested in discussing spiritual concerns. Waiting after the meeting had adjourned to meet any inquirers, I was left standing alone.

Zero response. "Well, that's that," I said. "A sharing group must not be what God wants." At the same time I felt foolish, humiliated and maybe a little angry.

The next day was a different story. To my delight, faculty members stopped me on the campus saying, "Hey, about that sharing group. I'm interested." We were off and going with a group of 12 people, including the Dean of the College and his wife, for a time of spiritual sharing that turned out to be one of my most precious experiences, and maybe their's too.

After leaving the college two years later because of Kay's physical deterioration and her desire to be near our children in Georgia, I received a message from the Dean saying that the group continued to function and was being blessed. I have always had the feeling that benefits for the participants of that group would extend beyond those two years we spent together. Only God knows, of course. But for me it was evidence of God's supernatural working, his taking me to the college to be blessed as well as to be a blessing to others. Of course my contact with students brought benefits too. But that is a matter I won't deal with here.

It all has to do with God's grace, this business of God's blessings. Anxiety doesn't triumph in times of uncertainty. God steps in. Experiences like this college one have shown me that God's grace is indeed real. I need not be troubled over any circumstance. Grace is God's provision for his continuing presence in our lives to set us free from all hindering forces. Our God, as Peter said, is "the God of all grace" (1 Peter 5:10).

Sharing Grace

One of the truisms of life is that we can best help someone who is experiencing a particular problem or setback when we ourselves have been through the same or similar circumstance. That is probably the most effective way of showing empathy and encouragement, since we know personally the suffering involved. Showing such care one for another is part of God's plan for our well-being—brothers and sisters in Christ coming to each other's aid to get through difficult times.

What does this have to do with grace? It is simply that as we grow in grace we are in a position to be conduits for God to dispense grace to others. We actually have a duty to do it, as seen in the instruction on caring for each other as members of the church body (1 Cor. 12:12–27). But I suspect it is the rare person who does it out of duty rather than out of compassion and love. Each of us has different strengths and abilities. The apostle Peter refers to them as God's gifts for use in helping one another:

> Each one should use whatever gift he has received to serve others, faithfully administering God's grace in its various forms. (1 Peter 4:10)

Did your eyes focus on the word "grace" in that passage? If not, you may want to go back and read it again. Part of our faithfulness to God is to share grace with others. We are told to be servants in this respect because the charge is to "serve others."

Look, the Lord can take care of our needs by zapping us in some miraculous way. And he apparently does that occasionally with some people. But he has chosen to deal with our problems primarily by using his children. I don't know why he follows that route, unless it is because he wants us to reap the joy of caring for one another. (And that, by the way, really does bring joy, both to the caregiver and the receiver.) But the fact is that it is a process he wants us to follow. Everybody caring for one another. I don't believe he wants us to do that if time, energy, money, or whatever permits. He is *expecting* us to do it. Period! You and I have God-given strengths (gifts) to do the job. Let's take his charge seriously of administering his grace to others. I will have a great deal more to say about this in the section on love.

The apostle Paul emphasized this theme as he instructed believers in Corinth who were undergoing troubling circumstances:

> Praise be to the God and Father of our Lord Jesus Christ, the Father of compassion and the God of all comfort, who comforts us in all our troubles, so that we can comfort those in any trouble with the comfort we ourselves have received from God. (2 Cor. 1:3–4)

In other words, God comforts us when we are hurting, and we in turn have the ability to comfort others, especially when the experiences take on similar characteristics. This is showing love in its grandest form, to "love each other deeply" and "faithfully administering God's grace in its various forms" (1 Peter 4:8–10). Grace encompasses love.

You can bet on my doing that when one of my friends loses his wife. I have been through it myself, so I know the suffering he is going through. We will talk together, pray together, cry together or just sit together. I can truly empathize with him because we share a common experience.

I am amazed as I watch this concept at work in my wife Deleta, who was gracious enough to marry me in 1999. She is able to show great empathy and render remarkable comfort to those grieving over the loss of a child because she herself experienced the death of a son, her first born from her previous marriage. At the age of twenty-one, Gregg was murdered on a Louisiana roadside while seeking help with his stalled car. Deleta's tender words now uplift bereaved mothers. How is it that she is so good at it? Because she went through the same kind of suffering. She now extends to others the comfort she received of God.

I would be remiss if I left the topic of "sharing grace" only on the note of caring for suffering people. Good things also happen to people, and those are times when we also need to get involved, to share happiness with them. The Bible tells us not only to cry with those who cry, but to rejoice with those who rejoice (Rom. 12:15). We tend to forget about this latter admonition. People who experience happy circumstances want others to share in their joy. The birth of a child, graduation from college, getting a job, winning an award, marriage, promotion, publishing a book, and a host of other experiences represent times when we would like friends to share in our happiness. We seem to have an innate desire for it. When we get involved, we are showing grace by being gracious. It strengthens bonds of friendship even further. It says, "I care."

How many times have we greatly rejoiced about some special happening in our lives only to be left celebrating it without the companionship of others. My late brother-in-law was a positive example for me. He was often there physically for happy events, such as my children's weddings, even to the extent of traveling great distances to share in their joy as well as mine. I think it was because of his good fortune to have parents whose example taught him to respect family and friends through his personal presence. It was one of his beautiful Italian customs which unfortunately I haven't seen much of in American culture.

We who haven't had the privilege of such a model when growing up have more difficulty being gracious. It isn't that we intentionally fail at it; we just seem to let opportunities slip by without thinking, or we balk financially if travel or a gift is involved, or if we are just too busy. The Spirit within us screams "Stop!" "Be gracious!" But we don't always listen.

Failure to share in one's happiness can turn that person's joy into sorrow. How do you suppose one reacts when family and friends show unconcern? Sadness and hurt. One's spirit is likely to be affected to the point of feeling abandoned. Nobody cares, is the message it sends. It creates an unhealthy situation which invites Satan's attacks to stir up sorrow and maybe even ill feelings. You might retort by saying, "So what do you want, a party every time you're happy? Grow up!" That is an overreaction that misses the point. Our aim is to be gracious on special occasions of joy which can be done even with a minimum of effort, such as a phone call when our physical presence isn't possible or even appropriate. How do you suppose the recipient of that call will feel? Pure delight over your graciousness.

We have an account in the Bible of Jesus attending a wedding. I doubt he was there just to turn water into wine. He must have wanted to honor the bride and bridegroom with his presence. He was always concerned about people. He fed the five thousand. He healed people's sick bodies and broken spirits. He sorrowed over his friend Lazarus. He protected his disciples from the storm. He received little children, perhaps placing them on his knees. Now it was a wedding! A joyous occasion for the newlyweds! And Jesus, being always gracious, was there honoring them.

Have you ever wondered about other celebrations Jesus attended and showed himself gracious, situations perhaps of lesser significance but at the same time of importance to the persons involved? Given his attitude toward people's feelings, he must have joined in on other happy events, although they are not recorded.

Anyway, many of us are familiar with the circumstance of family and friends coming together only at funerals. "What a pity that we get together only at such times as these," we say. "We ought to do it at happy events." Well, why don't we? God blesses people with special times of happiness. We acknowledge those blessings through our personal input, everybody rejoicing together over God's goodness.

Being gracious toward people in joyful situations requires effort on our part, something we aren't always willing to do. We don't view certain events in the lives of others as we do with the terminal act of death. "There will always be joyful occasions," we think, "so I can miss this wedding, or that anniversary." Have you ever attended the funeral of a family member or friend and thought about your negligence toward them while they were still alive?

Perhaps our challenge should be to do something right now to share in someone's joy. Even if there is no special occasion for it, do something to make them happy! Call or send a note to a family member, a friend, your pastor, the church pianist or organist, or whomever, to show your appreciation of them. And put it on your calendar as a reminder to do it toward someone maybe weekly. I promise you, the effect will be awesome. Just think about how you will feel if someone is gracious in that way to you. Oh yes, husbands and wives, complimenting each other at least once a week can do wonders for your marriage.

In case you have forgotten the topic of this chapter, it is *grace,* that is to say, accepting God's graciousness, and then being gracious to others by showing beauty and charm (Greek: *charis*). If this makes you uncomfortable, wait until you read Part III about your God-given responsibilities to love. But first, we go to Part II on faith. Stay with me for further blessings.

PART 2

- FAITH -

Introduction

Faith, used synonymously in the Bible with "believe," implies putting one's trust in God and his declarations. It is a most crucial word because it defines our relationship with our Creator both for eternal salvation and for maximizing a life of inner peace and joy on earth. It is what God desires for us. Just as an earthly father wants the very best for his children, so does God toward us (he actually calls us his sons and daughters), first in preserving our lives for eternity, and then in helping us enjoy life to the fullest on earth through intimate association with him. That relationship is enhanced by faith.

Faith is not divorced from that of our previous theme of *grace*. Accepting God's *grace* for salvation as well as for joy in living involves *faith*. For example, we believe what God says about forgiveness of our sins—past, present, and future—which is his grace provision for us to escape guilt and to rest with confidence and inner peace. It tells us he loves us in spite of our imperfections. That is grace, which we appropriate by faith.

Faith for the Christian follows grace. We act upon God's gracious provisions by believing (accepting) them. Listen to what Paul wrote the Roman believers:

> Therefore, since we have been justified through faith, we have peace with God through our Lord Jesus Christ, through whom we have gained access by *faith* into this *grace* in which we now stand. (emphases mine) (Rom. 5:1–2)

Throughout the New Testament is this connection between grace and faith repeated. They are sisters, as will be seen in the following chapter on faith.

CHAPTER 3

Exercising Faith

"Let us fix our eyes on Jesus, the author and perfecter of our faith."

Hebrews 12:2

Faith/belief for salvation is an issue one must deal with in order to initiate a relationship with God. It is a critical word because it defines our eternal destiny as well as a blossoming life of inner peace in everyday living. Inner peace, or resting in God's sovereignty, can be ours. It is important because we are beset with all kinds of happenings that cause turbulence in our lives. But we don't find inner peace without first settling the issue of faith for salvation.

Defining Faith for Salvation

Our journey of faith, then, begins with belief in Christ the Savior for salvation; it affects our eternal destiny. I take a few minutes to clarify this aspect of faith, should any readers be uncertain about where they will spend eternity.

The apostle Paul reminds us,

> For it is by grace you have been saved, through *faith.* (emphasis mine) (Eph. 2:8)

Another apostle, John, says,

> Yet to all who received him [Christ], to those who *believed* in his name, he gave the right to become children of God. (emphasis mine) (John 1:12)

("Received him" is John's way of saying "believed in him," as borne out by the second clause.)

Other New Testament writers talk about it too. The Bible is replete with teaching about this theme of salvation through faith.

This faith/belief in salvation goes well beyond mere intellectual assent. It demands our agreement with and submission to God's message on getting right with him. That is saving faith. This distinction between intellectual and saving faith is important. Not that the two are mutually exclusive, but I point this out should you be uncertain about your status. With which of the words do you identify? Many claim to believe in Christ as a historical figure, but that is not saving faith. It is head knowledge. Faith that saves involves acceptance of God's dictates about personal sinfulness and the need for forgiveness.

I like to distinguish between true and false belief by comparing two prepositions. Millions believe *about* Christ, but how many believe *in* him? This latter stance is one which answers the question, Why do I believe in him? It brings to the forefront the purpose of our belief. Are we believing *about* Christ, that is, that he once lived on earth, was a great teacher, or even that he is the Savior of the world in general but not ours in particular? Or are we believing *in* him for his redemptive act for us personally? That involves agreement with God about our sinfulness and need of redemption. It translates into seizing Christ's cross death for establishing union with him. Which preposition do you use with the word faith—*about* him or *in* him? Distinguishing between the two is crucial. James made reference to these differences when he said,

> You believe that there is one God. Good! Even the demons believe that—and shudder. (James 2:19)

He is saying that demons, although believing God exists and even that he has great power and authority, hardly believe in him for salvation. Demons aren't interested in salvation but rather in continuing their rebellion against God, as evidenced by their destructive activities against humanity.

I mentioned that salvation also requires submission to or agreement with God's message in Christ. Some people are too proud to do that in spite of God's easy offer of forgiveness. Or, they may reject the Bible's declaration of their sinfulness. They therefore must go without salvation. They see no need for it. They proceed through life thinking they are in control with no need to depend on God; that is to say, until they are devastated by some unexpected happening beyond their control. They ride high in life, boasting that they have need of nothing, until God brings them down. Some react negatively; they continue through life rejecting the Creator's loving offer of forgiveness through Christ. Others come to admit their insufficiency and look to Jesus for salvation. It is the attitude of submission (acknowledging dependence on Christ), that is linked to saving faith.

Living by Faith

Having taken the first step of faith for salvation, we proceed to walk in God's wisdom for transforming our earthly lives into a joyous experience. The rest of you readers, who have put your faith in Christ for salvation, perk up your ears! This further writing on faith is especially for you.

God wants you to have a life replete with peace and joy—blessings that come through understanding and acting upon his promises. That divine wisdom, if appropriated, will determine whether we live a ho-hum existence as Christians or whether we experience the dynamic, rewarding and fruitful life of which Jesus spoke.

The hurdle we face in living by faith is that, although trusting as little children, we tend to move away from a childlike trust as we become more aware of people's untrustworthiness. We become conditioned toward caution, and we carry it over to the spiritual. We learn to be analytical, to question, to demand proofs as conditional to belief. Seeing is believing, we say. We expect visible verification to support a truth. And so tends to be our attitude toward God.

The trouble is that it isn't God's way. We are to live by faith, not by sight, is Paul's message to first-century Christians (2 Cor. 5:7). People often say, "If only I could see a miracle, then I would have faith." I doubt it. If you can't believe without seeing, you probably will question a miracle performed before your very eyes. You will rationalize it away, just as some of the Jews must have done who, after witnessing the raising of Lazarus from the dead, went away unconvinced and even plotted to kill Jesus.

Jesus' own disciples had lessons to learn about miracles. They saw him perform plenty of them: a man cured of leprosy, the centurion's son healed, and many more. Yet when it came to believing that Christ could handle a storm on the lake threatening their personal safety, that was a different story. "Lord, save us! We're going to drown!" they screamed. What was Jesus' answer?

> You of little faith, why are you so afraid? (Matt. 8:26)

In another instance, they were worried for having forgotten to take food on their trip across the lake. How did Jesus respond?

> You of little faith, why are you talking among yourselves about having no bread? Do you still not understand? Don't you remember the five loaves for the five thousand, and how many basketfuls you gathered? Or the seven loaves for the four thousand, and how many basketfuls you gathered? (Matt. 16:8–10)

Prior to that, they had seen Jesus walk on water, and still they lacked faith in his control over all circumstances.

Faith is Trusting

Seeing does not always lead to believing. In its place is the need to simply believe God's declarations, to consider them trustworthy. And he has preserved his utterances in written form—the Bible. That holy revelation tells us:

> Faith comes from hearing the message, and the message is heard through the word of Christ. (Rom. 10:17)

In other words, we *depend* upon God to stand behind what he says. That is faith! It is not an exercise in futility, for God doesn't lie.

Dependency calls to mind Jesus' reference to children. Jesus wanted his disciples to understand that a trusting attitude is of utmost importance for a faith relationship with God.

> He called a little child and had him stand among them. And he said: 'I tell you the truth, unless you change and become like little children you will never enter the kingdom of heaven.' (Matt. 18:2–3)

Although faith for salvation seems to be the reference point here, an attitude of simple trust for overcoming life's problems is surely applicable as well.

At any rate, faith involves an attitude of total confidence, as seen in the complete trust little children have toward their mother, or when they believe what their father tells them simply because "Daddy said so." That puts a personal perspective on our relationship—sons and daughters walking in perfect faith with the Father. It is what God loves to see.

Jesus' Teachings

How do we put this into practice? Our dilemma comes when we look at some of the other statements Jesus made about faith. We become confused, because they don't prove to be true, we think. If you have faith, Jesus said, even in proportion to a little mustard seed, there is no end to the kind of things that will result (Matt. 17:20) (Luke 17:5–6). He used the example of moving mountains and trees, which obviously is not to be taken literally, since God has better things for us to do than to command the earth to move. The point is that faith is a force for wielding extraordinary happenings, even for producing miracles.

I want to explore the context of Jesus' statements about the mustard seed and moving mountains. It has to do with faith, but in a very specific context. We must not be guilty of using it to go off on a faith tangent, such as to try to perform healings wherever we go.

The incident had to do with the disciples' inability to heal a demon-possessed boy. Jesus was hard on them:

> How long shall I put up with you? Bring the boy here to me. (Matt. 17:17)

Can you catch Jesus' frustration with them? Time after time they lacked confidence in Jesus and in the power he made available to them.

To understand the demon incident involves looking at Jesus' charge seven chapters earlier, when he told his chosen twelve to perform specific acts of mercy, including casting out demons. Were they to follow those instructions even in the incident related to the demon-possessed boy in Matthew 17? We aren't told, but we can assume there was to be a carry-over—using the power of God to show mercy on people. Nevertheless, the disciples were powerless in that particular case. It may be that in the first incident recorded in Matthew 10 they had confidence and success in performing miracles; Jesus had just commissioned them to do it.

Seven chapters later, Jesus was not present to give them a direct charge to cast out the demon. (He came along later after they had bungled the job.) What was the problem then? They may have been depending on themselves instead of putting their faith in God. They had great power when Jesus sent them out previously. "Wow!" they must have thought. "We're really something that we could perform these miracles." Egos started to soar.

Acting with confidence in your own ability rather than in faith in God will do that to you.

Asking Jesus why they weren't able to heal the lad, they were told they lacked faith. That is why in the same breath Jesus told them about the little mustard seed. He had previously commissioned them to cast out demons. Now they needed simply to take him at his word, to proceed in faith in God's power, not their own. It was not a question of a great amount of faith. Jesus said they could do great things with just a speck of faith, as tiny as a mustard seed. But that faith had to be in God, not in themselves. Any ideas of self-grandeur would botch the job.

Can that happen to us? We have faith, for example, that we should pray over a sick person, and we do it successfully, resulting in someone's tumor disappearing, or in some other dramatic healing. It is like the disciples' great success recorded in Matthew 10. Then we work at duplicating it, but without success. God does heal, and sometimes he uses us as instruments of his healing. But he has not commissioned us, as he did with the Twelve, to go out and start healing every sick person we encounter. And what more, any notions of self-grandeur will surely work against us.

Our mistake is to assume that God intends for miracle workings to take place today to the same extent as in Jesus' time, and even as seen in the disciples' ministry after Jesus ascended to heaven. Why did those miracles take place then? They were a sign that this miracle worker, Jesus, was the promised Messiah, and that people should believe in him. John speaks about it:

> Jesus did many other miraculous signs in the presence of his disciples, which are not recorded in this book. But these are written that you may believe that Jesus is

> the Christ, the Son of God, and that by believing you may have life in his name. (John 20:30–31)

Of course Jesus healed out of mercy for those who were suffering. But John tells us he performed miracles so that people would believe he was the Messiah sent from God. Although Jesus had great compassion regarding people's physical wellness, he was more interested in their souls. Healings were Messiah's credentials. The Jews knew that from their Scriptures. Reading to them from the Old Testament, Jesus referred to a passage he connected with himself. He said that Isaiah's prophecy referred to him.

> The Spirit of the Lord is on me, because he has anointed me to preach good news to the poor. He has sent me to proclaim freedom to the prisoners, and recovery of sight for the blind, to release the oppressed, to proclaim the year of the Lord's favor. (Luke 4:18–19)

Messiah had come, and he had the power that accompanied his role as King over the kingdom he was destined to rule.

The problem of some people today is to regard that same miraculous power of the first century as belonging to them also. Distressed over people's suffering, they refer to Jesus commissioning the twelve to heal the sick and the oppressed, and then they act upon it without success. That leads to doubt and discouragement for them as well as for those with whom they deal. They are puzzled, because they thought they had faith. The absence of results may not have anything to do with lack of faith. Rather it is a presumption that Jesus' instructions to the twelve in that instance apply today.

Let's take a close look at the setting of those instructions. It was a very special one. First of all it specified that the disciples were to interact only with Jews. They were not to get involved with Gentiles. That is because the time had not yet come for non-Jews to be incorporated into God's plan of salvation. That would be revealed after the Cross, beginning with Peter at the house of Cornelius, the Roman centurion, an event which by the way opened the door for everyone to be accepted by God. It established all believers on earth, Jew and Gentile alike, as equal in Jesus Christ (Gal. 3:28).

Second, they were given a special message to proclaim, an exclusive Jewish message, that the Kingdom of Heaven was near. It was an appropriate announcement for the Jews of that era, whose religious orientation was that of Messiah coming to establish his rule. They were ready for deliverance from oppressive Roman subjugation. And word was out that Jesus was the actual Messiah, the one they were waiting for. Even after Jesus' resurrection were the apostles themselves holding to this kingdom issue, as seen by their question to Jesus:

> Are you at this time going to restore the kingdom to Israel? (Acts 1:6)

Yes, they acknowledged him as the Messiah, but they were still holding to Old Testament teaching about him in relation to an earthly kingdom pertaining to Israel as expressed in 2 Samuel, Chapter 7 and in several other Old Testament passages. It was natural for them to do that, since they didn't yet have God's full revelation. And Jesus didn't spell it out for them. They were not ready to understand it. The whole story unfolded after Jesus' return to heaven and the coming of the Holy Spirit to enlighten them.

The lesson for us is that the miracle workings of the Matthew 10 context must not necessarily be carried over as an automatic post-cross activity. Yes, I know that some insist this is not so, attributing lack of success to lack of faith. But even they will have to admit they are unable to perform miracles within the scope of the disciples' performance as in Matthew 10. We must be careful not to always grab hold of Jesus' instructions to the Twelve and to make them our own.

What were those instructions? A close look at them will show the foolhardiness of applying them to ourselves. First of all, he ordered the disciples to stay away from Gentiles and Samaritans. (They were to limit their ministry to Jews exclusively.) Second, they were to preach to those Jews that their long-awaited kingdom was about to come. Third, in addition to healing the sick in general, they were to restore people to health who were afflicted with leprosy. (None of this business of restricting healing to unseen internal illnesses.) And fourth and fifth, raising the dead and casting out evil spirits were to be done.

But that is not all. More instructions follow:

> Do not take along any gold or silver or copper in your belts; take no bag for the journey, or extra tunic, or sandals or a staff. (Matt. 10:9)

In other words, they were not to do what would be considered orderly planning—taking money, extra clothes, and making other preparation. They were to depend entirely on God to provide absolutely everything they needed.

Aside from isolated passages such as the above that are not intended for application apart from their contexts, the Bible does give us overwhelming instruction on faith.

To apply faith is to lean completely on God for direction rather than on our own devices. I know this through the Bible, but I have to activate it to make it work. It applies to any situation—future planning, suffering, ministering, or whatever.

Faith and Prayer

An important means of applying faith is through prayer. We see instances in which prayer is connected with healing the sick (James 5:14–15), building the spiritual life of believers (Phil. 1:9–11), and even things not particularly specified as per the following:

> And pray in the Spirit on all occasions with all kinds of prayers and requests. (Eph. 6:18)

The nature of prayer requests is not spelled out in its entirety. It seems to be left in part to the good sense of the petitioner, probably under the rubric of approaching the Father always in a spirit of submission to his will. That can certainly be supported by Jesus' prayer of agony in Gethsemane as he anticipated his Crucifixion:

> My Father, if it is possible, may this cup be taken from me. Yet not as I will, but as you will. (Matt. 26:39)

On the other hand, some people choose to emphasize strong faith as the most important ingredient in praying. They seem to measure prayer results in accord with faith, either theirs or someone else's. That way they can get off the hook if their prayers go unanswered. "We just didn't have enough faith," they say.

I have heard preachers say that it doesn't matter what your mountain is (referring to Mark's passage about moving mountains) (Mark 11:22). If you have faith, you can do anything, they claim. In other words, if you believe something strongly enough, your faith will make it happen. Yet we continually hear of events involving Christians supposedly strong in faith whose requests for healing are not answered. We even hear of parents withholding medical assistance from their children, resulting in the death of those innocent ones, and then attributing it to insufficient faith.

I do not minimize the importance of faith in prayer. Nor do I want to discourage anyone from praying for someone's healing. But we must recognize that there will always be things that God simply doesn't choose to happen in spite of our requests. It bears remembering that Paul, as strong in faith as he was, petitioned the Lord for personal healing without success (2 Cor. 12:9–10). God had other plans.

We may conclude that although God is capable and often wanting to perform miracles on our behalf, he will not be forced into it by our insistence that it come to pass. He is the potter, we are the clay, as Paul's letter to the Romans declares:

> But who are you, O man, to talk back to God? Shall what is formed say to him who formed it, 'Why did you make me like this?' Does not the potter have the right to make out of the same lump of clay some pottery for noble purposes and some for common use? (9:20–21)

We do not dictate to God in the name of faith.

I may ask God to come to my rescue on some troubling physical defect in my body (and the older I get, the more I find myself doing that), but he is the one to decide if reshaping is to take place. If you have trouble with that, you won't find the inner peace resulting from faith in a God who knows how best to respond. Instead, you are likely to become discouraged and disillusioned with God. I prefer the inner peace. How about you?

Returning to the Mark 11 passage (about faith and moving mountains), we would do well to understand that faith was never intended as an instrument to force God into action. That passage, as well as others that call for faith, must always be recognized within the framework of God's sovereignty and will.

Faith and Forgiveness

Another important consideration on prayer is Jesus' statement linking prayer and forgiveness. Mark's and Matthew's versions differ slightly in this regards.

> And when you stand praying, if you hold anything against anyone, forgive him, so that your Father in heaven may forgive you your sins. (Mark 11:25)

> For if you forgive men when they sin against you, your heavenly Father will also forgive you. But if you do not forgive men their sins, your Father will not forgive your sins. (Matt. 6:14–15)

On the surface the two statements seem to run contrary to the new covenant of grace instituted at the Cross. But God doesn't contradict himself. Interpretation must always be made in conjunction with other New Testament passages; otherwise, it destroys the substance of the whole plan of salvation through grace. It makes forgiveness from the Father conditional to our forgiving others, which is nothing less than a works-oriented salvation. It is certainly not new covenant teaching, one that is embedded in grace, unconditional in nature. And that is probably the underlying point in Jesus' statement. He was not speaking of the new covenant of grace. His listeners didn't have the slightest idea what the new covenant was, mainly because it had not yet been instituted through the Crucifixion (Luke

22:20). He was more likely referring to the characteristics of a faithful follower of God, something his Jewish listeners understood as a predominant feature of God's dealing with their ancestors as portrayed in their Holy Scriptures.

The idea is that God expects sincerity on the part of those who seek and follow him. One can't be sincere in accepting forgiveness while at the same time being unforgiving toward others. In fact, in another scenario Jesus underscored that truth in telling the parable of the unmerciful servant. The man was forgiven his huge debt but failed to forgive one of the guys who owed him.

> But when that servant went out, he found one of his fellow servants who owed him a hundred denarii. He grabbed him and began to choke him. 'Pay back what you owe me,' he demanded. (Matt. 18:28)

He then had the man thrown in jail in spite of his pleas for time to pay off the debt.

In contrast, we see a tender story of forgiveness in the Old Testament. Jacob portrayed it in his wish to his son Joseph—that he forgive his brothers for their wickedness toward him. (You will remember their cruelty in selling him into slavery.)

> I ask you to forgive your brothers the sins and the wrongs they committed in treating you so badly. Now please forgive the sins of the servants of the God of your father. (Gen. 50:17)

Joseph knew it was the right thing to do. But those last words of a dying father must have had a profound effect on Joseph. We see the emotional toll they took: when the message came to him, Joseph wept (v. 17).

Since we are in the post-cross era, under the new covenant of Christ, we have a clearer appreciation of the subject of sin and forgiveness. Let's remember what sins Christ paid for.

> When you were dead in your sins and in the uncircumcision of your sinful nature, God made you alive with Christ. He forgave us all our sins. (Col. 2:13)

The same sentiment is recorded in Colossians 3:13 as well as in Ephesians 4:32. That latter reference puts it this way:

> Be kind and compassionate to one another, forgiving each other, just as in Christ God forgave you.

In other words, new covenant teaching on forgiveness is explicit—we forgive others because we ourselves have been forgiven by God. We would be real ingrates if we did otherwise.

God's generosity through forgiveness is to be accepted by faith. It was revealed more clearly to the writers of the Bible after the Cross, because only then could it be understood in the context of salvation full and free, salvation through faith.

The trouble is that some Christians feel condemned when in their weakness they fail to practice forgiveness toward others. They see their error as one which Jesus condemns and consequently applies the chastisement of withholding his pardon, such as that spoken in the Matthew and Mark passages cited earlier. And without forgiveness they see themselves as totally out of favor with God, even resulting in loss of their salvation. Woe to them if suddenly they get killed in an automobile accident before they come to the point of confession. What it amounts to is a works-oriented salvation, one that fails to come to grips with the full gospel of grace. If you are still unsure about all of this, go back and reread Part I to review God's wonderful provision of grace.

I visited a church in my travels out of state where the pastor preached an entire sermon on forgiveness from the Matthew 6 passage. He played on the congregation's emotions by saying that their salvation depended on their forgiving others. "Don't argue with me!" he said. "Argue with God! What does the Bible say? It's as plain as can be. You won't be forgiven if you don't forgive."

This pastor preached from one single passage without attending to other biblical teaching on forgiveness and salvation. And judging from the burst of comments during the message of those around me—"That's what it says," "That's right," "Amen," "You tell 'em, brother," and the like—the congregation had not been trained to scrutinize Scripture as a whole, to compare a given passage with others, and to understand that passage within its particular context. The pastor was therefore gullible in forming doctrine from a single verse. I wondered whether it would be possible for me to discuss the sermon with him afterwards. He was standing at the door as I was leaving, beaming with pride over his "wonderful" discourse. I left without saying anything, but it was with sorrow and with prayers that God would help that church understand forgiveness through grace and faith.

Bad interpretation is often done with other passages too. Here is a classic one on faith versus works.

> What good is it, my brothers, if a man claims to have faith but has no deeds? Can such faith save him? (James 2:14)

Many see this verse as implying the need of deeds (works) for salvation. They fail to see that it speaks of a man who *claims* to have faith without showing evidence of its validity. It does not say that he *has* faith. That idea continues in the reference to demons believing (v. 19), which is hardly a belief for salvation.

I don't want to cite a listing of biblical passages that are often misinterpreted. The point I want to make is that we must not mistakenly look at a single passage without considering the context, either one immediately surrounding the passage or one embodied in the thrust of the entire New Testament. Otherwise, we are asking for discouragement and distrust of God, which will wreak havoc on our lives.

Let's keep Jesus' teaching on forgiveness in its proper context—that of instruction to people still under the Law, the old covenant. Jesus' intent was to help his listeners see their sinfulness and need of a Savior who would transform their lives. And that is exactly what took place upon initiation of the new covenant through his death.

Before closing this section, there is one more point to make on forgiveness. Let it be abundantly clear that God expects me to forgive you, and you to do likewise to me. It is a gross misinterpretation of Scripture to say we can hold grudges, for example, because God forgives us of all our sins. We are to be responsible in our dealings with one another (Col. 3:12–13).

There is no question that unforgiveness brings hurt to both parties. Pride as well as judgment of the other person as wrong deter forgiveness. A case in point is a rocky marriage relationship in which anger among spouses dominates and consequently brings pain and emotional stress. Peter's query relates to it. Asking Jesus how many times he should forgive someone, he was told there was no limit (Matt. 18:21–22). When both parties do that, it combats resentment and even feelings of retaliation. Forgiveness is enveloped in love, as verse 14 of the same Colossians passage states. No one in his right mind can be unforgiving and yet claim to operate out of love. Love is the defining characteristic of Christianity, as we will clearly see in the remaining three chapters. People who do not forgive have a love problem.

It isn't easy to forgive others who harm us in one way or another. The memory of the event embeds itself in our minds. The hurt often makes us angry and bitter. Enter faith! Allowing faith into the picture places the predicament in God's hands; it results in our relief as well as the ultimate resolving of the situation. After all, didn't God tell us to cast all our anxieties on him because he cares for us? (1 Peter 5:7).

Of course I have oversimplified the problem of forgiveness between people. Although forgiving doesn't compel a change of behavior on the part of the forgiven, it is hoped for. But whether or not it materializes, the concept of forgiving doesn't change. Jesus forgave us totally when we believed in him, and he continues to forgive in spite of our undesirable behavior. I should point out, however, that although he does that, he has provided instruction on correcting poor relationships. That is why the New Testament epistles were written—to teach us how to avoid making the same mistakes over and over again and hurting ourselves. Both parties, such as spouses, who are hurting must heed God's principles about relationships. But forgiving is to take precedence over change of behavior by the guilty party. That requires stamina. But it is always done in faith that God will give the offender the ability to change. Both parties will find it easier to do when letting God enter the picture through faith.

Faith Builders

At this juncture in our analysis of faith, let's think about how God blesses us with the end in mind of increasing our faith. There are times in every believer's life when God works on our behalf in spite of our lack of faith. That may happen when God does good things but receives no recognition from us of his interaction. Failure to give him credit is a basic problem of human nature. We go about our busy lives thinking that a turn for the better in life was just coincidence. "How lucky," we say. But God understands our lack of sensitivity of his interventions. So he has to call our attention to different happenings in our lives, sometimes doing it in unusual ways, to teach us of his goodness and to increase our faith in him.

My wife Deleta has seen God's patience with her in this regard. The church she attended years ago put out a monthly newsletter to encourage its members to walk in faith. In one issue, several people told their story about how God had spoken to them. (Deleta's interpretation as a neophyte in these matters was that he had talked to them orally.) Here was her reaction.

> I became a very angry lady. I told God how mad I was. He talks to others but not to me. What else I said I don't remember, but I know I cried. I felt left out. I was in for a big surprise that night. I remember waking up with the thought pounding in my head, 'But don't you remember when you were troubled about the excessive overtime demands of your job? You had little time to spend with your family, so I found you that new job at the YWCA.' I fell back to sleep only to be awakened with another thought. 'Don't you remember when I provided the money you needed last year when you were in a financial pinch? And it was the

> exact amount you needed to boot.' I fell asleep again, only to be awakened with another 'Don't you remember . . .?' The process went on the entire next day, calling to mind different occasions when God had involved himself with my needs.
>
> I was guilty of having utterly failed to recognize his intervention. It turned out to be a real faith builder—my Heavenly Father calling to my mind his tenderness and love which I had been guilty of not recognizing. And I'm no longer naive to think that his communication has to be vocal. He spoke to me quietly by bringing to mind his faithfulness.

Deleta learned that God builds faith through different circumstances, even though at the time they occurred she wasn't aware of his involvement. I suppose we all share that experience in one way or another. Unfortunately, we are slow learners. But God is patient. He doesn't blow his top, but rather helps us grow in trust toward him. Is that not characteristic of a loving heavenly Father? He doesn't get angry, nor does he belittle us and call us stupid. He just carries on with patience, kindness and love, knowing that at some point we will recognize his goodness.

Think about it! How many times have you had good things happen to you for which you didn't give God the credit? We might all do well to reflect on events in our lives to discover God's tender care. Ask God to help you remember. In fact, you may want to take time at the end of the day to rehearse the circumstances in which God was involved, and to give him praise. Increased awareness of his involvement is a faith builder. It tells you that he is always in control, and that he cares particularly about you. Then give thanks, much thanks, to a gracious and caring Heavenly Father.

A word of caution is due here. As with grace, faith is a process we grow in. Don't think that you are going to become a giant of faith instantly. Paul commended Thessalonian believers for their *growth* in faith (2 Thess. 1:3). He also encouraged those in Ephesus with a similar challenge:

> That Christ may dwell in your hearts through faith. (Eph. 3:17)

He is not talking about people coming to grips with faith for salvation. The recipients of Paul's letters to the Thessalonians and Ephesians were Christians; they had already put their faith in Christ for salvation. Now they were being commended for their growth in faith. Both groups were being encouraged to make faith a part of their daily lives, to grow in it.

Tests of Faith

Although I have learned to lean on God through a multitude of experiences, some good and some bad, I know my faith yet remains small. I am still vulnerable to faithlessness. I am not just talking about trusting God in things of temporary significance, such as loss of a job, or destruction of material possessions as through fire or a car wreck, as bitter as those situations are. Think about really big happenings! I mean, will you walk in faith if your child dies? A dear brother in Christ had his thirteen-year-old son die in his arms on the way to the hospital. He and his wife were devastated. In church the next Sunday, as Deleta approached the mother to offer comfort, she faced a woman who, albeit with tears streaming down her cheeks, was holding fast to God's trustworthiness. She didn't understand why her son was taken. Who can in a situation such as that? But she maintained faith in God's wisdom and sovereignty. Maybe God foresaw and decided to prevent some devastating experience to come upon the boy later in his life. Maybe some unfortunate things would have happened to other people had the boy remained alive. We can come up with all kinds of suppositions, but they will not satisfy our questioning why the tragedy had to happen. We don't know the reasons. The best we can do is to follow the advice of Thomas à Kempis who wrestled with similar problems and said, "Get used to knowing less than God."[1]

How about if your spouse is diagnosed with a terminal illness? (And guess who will be the caregiver.) What if your father or mother or other family member gets killed? What if a loved one ends up with a crippling disease? These are real tests of faith, and unfortunately they happen. When they find us as their target, is it unfair? Do we shake our fists at God and blame him?

We have untold examples in the Bible of suffering by God-fearing people: Joseph, sold into slavery, and later unjustly sentenced to prison; Daniel, thrown to the lions in Babylon; Job, afflicted in horrible ways by Satan; John the Baptist, beheaded; Stephen, stoned to death; and the Old Testament prophets, enduring sufferings that defy imagination, as referred to by the writer of Hebrews:

> They were stoned; they were sawed in two; they were put to death by the sword. They went about in sheepskins and goatskins, destitute, persecuted and mistreated—the world was not worthy of them. They wandered in deserts and mountains, and in caves and holes in the ground. (Heb. 11:37–38)

But when it comes to us, we don't understand why God allows us to suffer. Our favorite question is "Why?" Our favorite declaration is "Unfair!"

I don't mean to put a guilt trip on you. We all question God at one time or another and we even think we know how and when God should solve our problems. I have to catch myself from doing that from time to time. Even the psalmist had trouble understanding why God seemed to be distancing himself. "Why have you forgotten me?" he asked (Ps. 42:9). But it was a temporary state. Yes, he was disheartened, but he always came back to reality about a trustworthy Lord.

> Why are you downcast, O my soul? Why so disturbed within me? Put your hope in God, for I will yet praise him, my Savior and my God. (Ps .42:11)

I was put to this test in caring for my late wife. Let me tell you what suffering is. Here was a woman with a rare terminal disease called PSP (Progressive Supranuclear Palsy) causing a multitude of heartaches over a ten-year period. Hers was unbelievable suffering: disorientation, loss of muscular control, loss of speech, choking, feeding tube, incontinence, diapers, catheter tube, breathing difficulty, oxygen mask, pain, screaming, pneumonia. Yet in all that time—trust. "He takes care of me," she uttered in a faint, nearly incomprehensible whisper.

Emotional hurt for family and close friends always accompanies the physical suffering of the loved one. How often did husband and children step out of the room with faces awash in tears. Then the sleepless nights, loss of appetite, the stress, the depression, the breakdown in health of the caregiver husband. Ten years of crying out to God for mercy. I could identify with the psalmist when he said:

> I am worn out from groaning.; all night long I flood my bed with weeping and drench my couch with tears. (Ps. 6:6)

It is not unparalleled. I remind you of the famous scriptural passage on faith previously cited. It tells us about those of old who were tortured, flogged, stoned, killed by the sword, and even sawed in two (Heb. 11:35–37). Can you imagine that? Sawed in two. It makes me cringe just to think about it. And then there was Job, perhaps the ultimate example of faith in adversity. Yet none of them gave up on God. They knew that this short sojourn on earth was not to be compared with the eternity God had in store for them.

My personal suffering over the extended illness and eventual death of my wife caused me to come to grips with the reality of faith. "Okay Ted," I said to myself. "Are you going to practice faith or just talk about it?" "Is it going to be real or just information?" The latter is knowledge drilled into me by preachers, Bible teachers, and even the Bible itself through my reading, study and memorization. *Applying* faith is something entirely different. At this dramatic time it meant coming to grips with my helplessness in controlling the situation. After all, who determines when death comes and all the suffering preceding it? The disease afflicting my wife was horrendous in the toll it took on her. God could have healed her, and many prayers were offered to that end. But he said no! It was time for her to join him in heaven.

Accepting that decision became more than an intellectual exercise. It was heart-induced trust, a dedication to belief that God cares and is doing what he deems best. In my helplessness I became aware, more than ever before, that God was in control. It gave me the necessary resources with which to cope. No, I didn't understand God's rationale in withhold healing and restoration. I didn't like the outcome. But still there was peace, which told me that God understands my perplexity and discomfort. "Just don't give up on me, Ted," was the message pounding in my ears.

"You'll understand completely after you've finished your brief sojourn on earth. Trust me!"

We can be challenged by Job who, having undergone untold physical suffering (painful sores) and mental duress (death of his children, loss of all material possessions, and false accusation by "friends"), was yet able to say, "Though he slay me, yet will I trust in him." Besides that, he had to put up with a wife who was fed up with it all and told him to curse God and die! (Job 2:9).

Be strong in faith! says the writer of Hebrews, "so that you will not grow weary and lose heart" (Heb. 12:3). He knew that times would come when we would be especially vulnerable to Satan's attacks. No matter how extraordinary the situation, we must cling to God in faith, so that we will not "grow weary and lose heart."

We are the creation of an awesome God whom we sometimes fail to acknowledge as the Almighty, the Ruler of the Universe, the All Wise, the All Knowing, and the All Powerful. In spite of his great faith, Job took this Everlasting Being to task for what he thought was undeserved suffering. God in turn posed a number of questions to remind him of the Almighty's sovereignty. Look at what he said to Job:

> Where were you when I laid the earth's foundation? Tell me if you understand. Who marked off its dimensions? Surely you know! Who stretched a measuring line across it? On what were its footings set, or who laid its cornerstone—while the morning stars sang together and all the angels shouted for joy? Who shut up the sea behind doors when it burst forth from the womb, when I made the clouds its garment and wrapped it in thick darkness, when I fixed limits for it and set its doors and bars in place, when I said, 'This far you may come and no farther; here is where your proud waves halt?' Have you ever given orders to the

> morning, or shown the dawn its place? Have you journeyed to the springs of the sea or walked in the recesses of the deep? Have the gates of death been shown to you? Have you seen the gates of the shadow of death? Have you comprehended the vast expanses of the earth? Tell me, if you know all this? (Job 38:4–18)

Having been reminded of the great gulf between the wisdom of the Creator and that of the created, Job came to his senses and responded,

> I am unworthy—how can I reply to you? I put my hand over my mouth. (Job 40:4)

So it was with me as I watched my wife wither away. Suffering and death test one's faith. They forced me to recognize God's omnipotence and my dependence on him. I could only repeat Job's words: "I am unworthy—how can I reply to you?"

Faith and Doubt

In the foregoing discussion I have suggested some approaches to understanding faith and growing in it. Earlier I also suggested the reality of doubt, the opposite of faith, which I believe is realistic in recognition of our human limitations to trust. That topic deserves further discussion.

Let's face it. We have our weak moments. We doubt. I do. You do. Doubt often takes the form of rationalization, which is good to some extent, because reasoning is a starting point for initial belief for salvation as we admit our sinfulness. We see sense in the Bible's teaching on the necessity of pardon, and we accept the gospel story of God's forgiveness. But after that, reason tends to get in the way of faith, especially in times of extraordinary suffering. Some people go even further as they wonder if their belief is sustainable, perchance out of fear of receiving God's declarations too simplistically.

I suspect such was the case with Judas, whose eventual doubt about the validity of Christ as the long-awaited Messiah resulted in his tragic suicide. But he wasn't the only one of Jesus' disciples who doubted. Peter must have wondered whether his faith was justified when he saw Jesus being arrested. Aren't you one of his disciples? they asked him. "I am not," he answered (John 18:17). Wow! Peter saying that, after all he went through with Jesus? Then there was doubting Thomas, that great example of faithlessness that has become a part of our vocabulary.

Mark's gospel recounts the story of Peter, James, and John as they accompanied Jesus to join the other disciples who at that very moment were struggling to resolve the matter of healing the boy (Mark 9:14). It is a development not included in the Matthew account, but it is important in the story of doubt that afflicts all of us. Let's review the incident to see what more can be extracted from it. The boy's father told Jesus:

> Teacher, I brought you my son, who is possessed by a spirit that has robbed him of speech. Whenever it seizes him, it throws him to the ground. He foams at the mouth, gnashes his teeth and becomes rigid. I asked your disciples to drive out the spirit, but they could not . . . But if you can do anything, take pity on us and help us. (Mark 9:17–18, 22)

Jesus responded saying that everything is possible for him who believes. The father replied with an amazing statement:

> I do believe: help me overcome my unbelief! (v. 24)

Now what in the world does that mean? He believed but yet he didn't? It was an honest confession of both belief and doubt on the part of the boy's father. Perhaps better stated, it was a desire to believe but also beset by confusion and uncertainty, which happens with us too, by the way. Yet it didn't interfere with Jesus healing the boy. Admission of confusion or doubt is healthy; it recognizes our limitations. There is no sense feeling guilty about it. It is being honest with God. And he doesn't clobber us for doubting; rather, he values honesty.

The apostles acknowledged their spiritual weakness when they asked Jesus to increase their faith (Luke 17:5). They knew through Jesus' preaching that people were to have faith, and in the epistles they wrote later they encouraged their readers to grow in faith.

Growing in faith may have something to do with experience in life, with accumulating wisdom, which has its connection with age. I must confess that I doubted more in my younger years compared to now. Maybe it is a resignation to things I know I can't change, like having a body whose parts are functioning more imperfectly than they were fifty years ago. It makes for a greater awareness of the temporary nature of our stay in this world.

Could that be typical of senior citizens in giving them a greater disposition toward faith? I do find elderly Christians talking more about faith than do young people. It seems to make sense, since they have experienced so much more. No wonder the Bible associates wisdom with our elders. Wisdom and faith seem to accompany each other.

God's Omnipresence

I want to take this topic of faith, and perhaps doubting, one step further. It has to do with God's omnipresence, a divine characteristic we often fail to recognize, unfortunately to our detriment. First of all, remembering that God is everywhere, including holding our hand so to speak, I see his omnipresence having a positive impact on our prayer life. Let me give a personal example.

Although I knew God always listened to me, I failed to appreciate the fact of his presence while I prayed. I somehow missed the reality of God living within me, as if he were standing before or beside me—both of us communing together. I knew the scripture passage that taught that Jesus would be with me always (Matt. 28:20), that he and the Father would make their home in me (John 14:23), and that the Holy Spirit would live in me (John 14:16–18). But somehow I failed to connect it with the intimacy of prayer. Why does that matter? Because when I pray, I have a helper in the third person of the trinity, the Holy Spirit. Look at how Paul explains it.

> The Spirit helps us in our weakness. We do not know what we ought to pray for, but the Spirit himself intercedes for us with groans that words cannot express. And he who searches our hearts knows the mind of the Spirit, because the Spirit intercedes for the saints in accordance with God's will. (Rom. 8:26–27)

Having a sense of God's nearness (omnipresence) is like having his arms around me in a caring embrace. It tells me I am wanted and loved, which gives me faith that he will help me in one way or another. It makes me more cognizant of his presence in all of life's experiences. I connect with him. God is not some impersonal being who is off in space somewhere. He is within us. Ponder the implications.

I am reminded of a great hymn of C. Austin Miles entitled *In the Garden*, whose gentle words speak so tenderly: "He walks with me and he talks with me, and he tells me I am his own. And the joy we share as we tarry there, none other has ever known." God in us. That is what the apostle John surely meant when he quoted Jesus as saying,

> If anyone loves me, he will obey my teaching. My Father will love him, and we will come to him and make our home with him. (John 14:23)

God making his home with us. My wife Deleta saw that truth after the fact, but now her faith is more attuned to God's omnipresence in current happenings. I think that is what the psalmist was about when he said,

> If I go up to the heavens, you are there: if I make my bed in the depths, you are there. If I rise on the wings of the dawn, if I settle on the far side of the sea, even there your hand will guide me, your right hand will hold me fast. (Ps. 139:8–10)

There is yet another aspect to my consideration of faith and God's omnipresence or proximity. It has a salutary effect on the way I control my daily life. When I am more conscious of our Lord's continual presence I am pressed toward greater care in governing my behavior. It makes me realize that such behaviors as anger, bitterness, slander, and malice toward people, for example, affect God (Eph. 4:31). How is that so? Scripture tells us that the Holy Spirit actually grieves over our negative conduct (Eph. 4:30). I don't suppose it is a matter of him saying, "Look at what you are doing. You are hurting me." If he is hurt, he is likely to be so more out of grief and concern *for us*, not for himself, knowing that our negative ways harm us, to say nothing of how they affect those around us.

God is interested in our welfare, as we have seen in the Holy Spirit interceding for us with groans that can't be expressed in words (Rom. 8:26). God loves his children, and is grieved when we hurt ourselves and others too, just as we as earthly parents are saddened when our own children get involved in things that harm them.

Other sins are found among us that are not visibly expressed. We think they are secret sins, like lust, for example, because it is not visible to others but is hidden within the confines of our minds. But do we face the reality that those "secret sins" are not secret at all? The Father, Son, and Holy Spirit living within us see them and are affected by them. If God cries, he must weep at our thoughtlessness.

You might respond, "Why should he care? It's my life. If I do something to hurt myself, *I* will put up with the consequences." I remind you that God, being the loving Father, is concerned about any harm we might do to ourselves as well as the repercussions it may have on others. Brothers and sisters in Christ, he is a part of us! He actually lives within us! Our awareness of that miraculous presence should induce us toward greater self-control as we face our human frailties. It renders to us the joy that comes from knowing we truly live in intimate companionship with a very forgiving and loving Lord. It is faith in action.

What Can We Do?

Where do we go from here? How do we apply faith to our lives? I find myself lacking it when I have an attitude problem about who is in control. Of course, the ideal is to recognize God being behind every situation, but my practicing it, that is, really believing it, is another matter. So I want to emphasize that the application of faith is a reality that goes beyond mere knowledge.

I have often wondered about the category Jesus would have placed me in had I been among his listening audience back in the first century. You may remember that with some people "he was amazed at their lack of faith" (Mark. 6:6), while with others he was moved by their simple yet total trust. Among the former were Jews who ridiculed him and even tried to stone him to death. They just couldn't come to grips with him being the sent one of God. In contrast, among those with a firm belief was the sick woman who sneaked behind him to touch his clothes (Matt. 9:21). She didn't harangue him for healing. Just to touch his garment was all she needed.

Luke adds more detail to this tender story by citing Jesus' awareness of the touch.

> Then the woman, seeing that she could not go unnoticed, came trembling and fell at his feet. In the presence of all the people, she told why she had touched him and how she had been instantly healed. (Luke 8:47)

The result of her faith was not only her personal healing; it was a witness to all the onlookers of the power of faith exhibited through a mere touch. Think about it. The woman believed she would be healed simply by touching Jesus' clothes. And she was right. She put her belief into action.

Similar episodes of faith are recorded regarding the paralytic, two blind men, and the daughter of the Canaanite woman. You can find those events in Matthew, Chapters 9 and 15. But perhaps the most striking example of unquestioning trust was that of the Roman centurion.

When Jesus had entered Capernaum, a centurion came to him, asking for help.

> 'My servant lies at home paralyzed and in terrible suffering.' Jesus said to him, 'I will go and heal him.' 'The centurion replied, 'Lord, I do not deserve to have you come under my roof. But just say the word, and my servant will be healed. For I myself am a man under authority, with soldiers under me. I tell this one, Go, and he goes; and that one, Come, and he comes. I say to my servant, Do this, and he does it.' When Jesus heard this, he was astonished and said to those following him, 'I tell you the truth, I have not found anyone in Israel with such great faith.' (Matt. 8:5–10)

Here we learn of the centurion's servant who was undergoing great physical pain. The centurion exhibited supreme faith by asking only for Jesus to speak a word in order for healing to take place. And his servant wasn't even present at the time. Embedded in his attitude was that of great respect for Jesus' authority. He deemed it so powerful that just a word by Jesus would be effective even across distance. He also must have had great humility in approaching Jesus, since his military status put him in a position of authority. (Begging for help was probably not a part of his usual behavior.) But for some reason he recognized Jesus as someone special, someone sent by God with power to do something for his servant that no one else could do.

I suggest that in his two attitudes—respect for Jesus' authority and a humble spirit—lies the key to faith. It amounts to a complete abandonment of self by putting oneself in God's hands. It asks for an attitude of unquestioning belief, just as was had by the sick woman and the Roman centurion. Faith was evidenced by their simplistic attitudes of touching Jesus' clothes and merely asking the Master to say the word for the person not even present to be healed.

The test of faith, however, is when we continue believing God as trustworthy even though the outcome may not be to our liking. The sick woman and the centurion got positive responses. We may also, but then we may not. The latter is hard to take, but God would have us accept a no response with a continuation of faith. Christians full of faith stand firm in their trust no matter whether God's response is contrary to their hopes. That is an attitude that can be ours as we seek God to develop it in us. It is not something to be completed in one fell swoop. Faithless questioning stubbornly clings to our minds; old habits don't disappear over night.

Negative situations abound for us in life, and we need faith to combat them. Our adversary is constantly throwing them at us for our hurt. That is why Paul instructs us to:

> Take up the shield of faith, with which you can extinguish all the flaming arrows of the evil one. (Eph. 6:16)

Faith is an important defensive measure. It helps us stand firm against Satan's attacks. But it is also an offensive weapon, as Paul tells the Thessalonians,

> We continually remember before our God and Father your work produced by faith. (1 Thess. 1:3)

What was that *work*? Paul explains:

> The Lord's message rang out from you . . . your faith in God has become known everywhere. (1 Thess. 1:8)

In all their activity, the Thessalonian Christians exhibited the element of faith and therefore, according to Paul, "became a model to all the believers" (v. 7). Undoubtedly, it also came into play with evangelism. It must have touched the lives of many nonbelievers, since the spreading of the gospel was always an integral part of the early church's ministry.

Faith Abused

People seem to have a penchant for taking something intended for their good and turning it into something destructive. I see that being done today through a religious movement that frightens me. It is the so-called health and wealth gospel, or prosperity gospel, which I hope to convince you to be a concept concocted by men, not by God. As we have seen in Chapter One on Grace, manmade ideas with a flavor of religiosity are extremely dangerous. Jesus condemned them.

Proponents of this movement herald it as an expression of faith which will result in our physical wellness and material prosperity. I discuss this movement here because of the error of relating it to faith, but also because of the damaging effect it wields on many who embrace it as well as on the world's image of Christianity.

A disturbing statement made by its proponents is that God never intended that we be sick or poor. That message is not brand new. It must have existed years ago, although not to the extent of its popularity today. I say that because during my college days of the 1950s, a fellow student, whom I viewed as super spiritual because he always had a serious look on his face, chided me for having the flu. "Why would you allow yourself to get sick?" he asked, implying that a reliance on the Holy Spirit would deter illness. What more, he connected it with sin in my life, saying, "Ted, if you would get right with the Lord, you wouldn't be suffering with that flu." I couldn't help but equate him with Job's "comforters."

The problem we face with the health and wealth message is the same we face with other human ideas we connect with religion. It produces a great deal of guilt and frustration on the part of those who embrace it but then are not blessed with its promised results. They feel that way because they are led to believe that the absence of blessing of both health and wealth is a consequence of their lack of faith. It is failing to take advantage of God's blessings, they say. The worst scenario is their turning from God, deeming him untrustworthy when the proposed benefits are not received.

The wealth component of this faith phenomenon attracts a vast audience, perhaps one far greater than those looking for healing. Wealth commands people's attention, because when it comes to getting rich, people really tend to perk up their ears. Point out a few Bible verses that seem to refer to blessings of wealth awaiting them, and bingo, you have them hooked.

We see a typical source of error in this approach—failure to understand biblical passages in their proper context; that is to say, context in tune with the overall teaching of the Bible. Plucking verses out of the Old Testament such as: Proverbs 8:18–21, Psalm 1:3; Psalm 112:1–3; and, Joshua 1:8—all of which are supposed to imply that God bestows wealth on those who follow him—is hardly an appropriate means of establishing a doctrine.[2] Yes, God may choose to bless some with financial prosperity, but he doesn't give license to establish it as normative. God decides who, if any, is to be made rich. And I doubt the correctness of asking him for wealth, unless you are going to pluck out of Scripture some obscure passage like the recently made popular "prayer of Jabez" (1 Chron. 4:9–10) and read into it an expected blessing.

Another thing that greatly distresses me about faith for material gain is that the health and wealth preachers are cleaning up on their audiences to their own financial prosperity. It greatly troubles me because of its harmful reflection on the Gospel of Christ. You will recall that "gospel" means good news. It is not good news when we see it mixed with ripping people off in the name of spirituality.

I am amazed at the gullibility of people who support these guys who are living high on the hog with their million-dollar mansions, expensive automobiles, and the rest of their lavish life styles. If God weeps, he must be shedding tears over those who make a business out of preaching the gospel. They are proclaiming God's free gift and getting rich on it. It is as if they are saying, "Here's God's free gift of salvation for you. But I'm charging you for it." If that is not a contradiction, I don't know what is.

In contrast, a man in Louisiana is preaching the Word without asking for a dime. His financial support is his Social Security check and his meager retirement benefits. His is an interesting story.

Having conducted highly acclaimed Bible classes in Baton Rouge, Nick was approached by a class member who suggested he teach the Bible on radio. He declined because of his desire to follow the apostle Paul's example in ministry and was uncomfortable having to appeal to his listeners for funds to pay for air time. He was then asked if he would reconsider if class members would provide funds to kick off such an effort. He agreed and class members responded with enough pledges to cover six months of radio time.

The broadcasts quickly became self-supporting. Out of appreciation for the solid expository teaching they were hearing, listeners began making their own contributions. But the beauty of it is that they did it without being asked. Never was there an appeal for money. No one ever received a salary or any kind of payment for services. This has been going on for 17 years. Yes, Nick is experiencing prosperity, but it is not financial. He is prospering by seeing people blessed through careful and clear presentation of the Word of God.

That is what I consider practicing true grace—giving biblical instruction without asking for anything in return. Or is the idea of making the gospel freely available something that is just characteristic of God?

I can't help but recall the apostle Paul's attitude in all of this. Look at what he said:

> What is my reward? Just this, that in preaching the gospel I may offer it free of charge. (1 Cor. 9:18)

Paul worked to support himself (1 Cor. 9). When failing to earn enough funds, he accepted financial help, but only to meet his bare needs. And Barnabas followed suit (v. 6).

I point out Paul's attitude toward ministering under financial hardship as a contrasting example to those who accumulate wealth in the name of the Lord. I am not proposing that people in the professional ministry support themselves in extra jobs (although some do that under personal conviction). Paul was certainly unique. He didn't require others to emulate him on money matters, because he knew that compensation was due those who give themselves to the work of the ministry. He knew they may have families to support, or perhaps have other financial obligations to meet.

There is little doubt that Paul was different. He probably distinguished himself from most others in the ministry. Although he defended the right to receive material support, he surrendered that right so as not to hinder the gospel (1 Cor. 9:12).

Getting rich on the gospel probably has been a consuming evil throughout the ages. It was a problem with the start up of Christianity 2,000 years ago, as we see in Paul's account to Timothy (1 Tim. 6:3–11) about teachers "who think that godliness is a means to financial gain" (v. 5). Paul reminded him,

> People who want to get rich fall into temptation and a trap and into many foolish and harmful desires. (v. 9)

It must have really bothered Paul, as evidenced by his statement:

> Unlike so many, we do not peddle the word of God for profit. (2 Cor. 2:17)

Great caution must be taken in mixing the gospel with money matters.

But what about the health part of the prosperity gospel? Like its wealth component, it misuses scripture by restricting itself to verses that seem to endorse its viewpoint (Ex. 23:25; Ps. 103:3–5; and certain New Testament references on believing and receiving). The idea that God doesn't want us to be sick or even die early sounds wonderful; it reinforces ideas about a compassionate and merciful Father. But God will not be forced into performance based on a mistaken understanding of faith.

Note that three of Paul's fellow workers in the ministry got sick. And it wasn't just a matter of a head cold. Epaphroditus almost died (Phil. 2:26–27), Trophimus had to be left behind because of illness (2 Tim. 4:20), and Timothy suffered recurring bouts of sickness (1 Tim. 5:23). If Paul's thorn in the flesh was a physical malady, we can add him to the list (2 Cor. 12:7).

In place of this prosperity gospel, what should be our guiding principle? It should be to walk in faith and love without even thinking about getting anything materially from God in return. It was that same message Paul had for first-century believers who were confused about other matters, such as inflicting manmade rules on people. Paul made it clear that what really counted was to walk in faith and love (Gal. 5:6). The purpose of that walk is the intimacy it develops with God. It is a love relationship that God wants us to have with him. Knowing the reality of faith and love keeps us on track with a life of *spiritual* health and wealth.

The Bible speaks a great deal about faith. But to jump on it as a magic word for insuring prosperity is not the way the Bible tells us to exercise faith. Put on faith! God urges. The end product, however, is nonmaterial. It is the practice of love (1 Thess. 5:8). Part III will tell you about love, love in action, our third great word of the Bible. Read on to learn from it.

PART 3

- LOVE -

Introduction

We must now investigate the phenomenon of love as we continue to develop our understanding of Christianity for the purpose of reaping its full benefits. Like grace and faith, love doesn't stand alone. All three are interrelated as they involve our Christian experience, first in coming to understand God's goodness outpoured toward us in making us his children, and then in developing an intimate relationship with him in daily living, all to the benefit of our joy.

It is appropriate to deal with the subject of love after having discussed faith. Paul said,

> If I have a faith that can move mountains, but have not love, I am nothing. (1 Cor. 13:2)

That translates to love's importance above everything else. That doesn't minimize the significance of grace and faith. Love emanates from them. It is spurred on when we attune ourselves toward God's gracious acts and continual blessings. As I view my Christian life in progress I see that my love is in proportion to the degree to which I apply grace and faith. As the Bible tells us that love is the greatest of all spiritual strengths (1 Cor. 3:13), it maintains a unity or interconnection between all three words

The subject of love encompasses a number of areas: God's love in providing salvation, his show of love in our daily affairs, our love toward him in return, and his command that we love others. I will touch on all of these, but will concentrate on love in relation to *our* love toward God and toward people. I will suggest some practical steps in regard to the growth of that love. Loving people is broken down into; (1) loving Christians (Chapter 5); and, (2) loving all people (Chapter 6). But first, growing in love for God.

CHAPTER 4

Loving God

"Love the Lord your God with all your heart and with all your soul and with all your mind."

Matthew 22:37

Our stature as Christians is evidenced by our love for God. C. S. Lewis believed that people's spiritual health is in direct proportion to that love. [1] In other words, the more we grow in loving God, the more we thrive spiritually. But pity those whose love for God goes little beyond their salvation experience. They have been given spiritual birth but lack closeness with the one who brought about new life. Their view of him tends to be subjugated to ideas of goodness and truth not much different from those of non-Christians. Tozer reflects on this phenomenon by saying that for many, loving God is merely an ideal or a principle.[2] There is little or no personal experience in such a relationship. That makes loving God difficult.

The test of true love is not merely to acknowledge it as a nice moral principle but to make it a part of our lives, to practice it. People who think they are spiritual but don't practice love have missed out on the most important aspect of Christianity. They may have great knowledge, possess several spiritual gifts, and perform various acts of benevolence, but if they lack love for God they have missed the boat regarding God's main expectation, indeed blessing, of them. That is why Scripture declares that among all spiritual signs "the greatest of these is love" (1 Cor. 13:13).

KNOWLEDGE VERSUS EXPERIENCE

Our spiritual journey in love begins with a knowledge-based acceptance of God's declaration on the subject. But then it must become experiential. For example, we learn from Scripture that God's love for us is unconditional; he loves us no matter how we may err in thought or deed. Consider Paul's words:

> Who shall separate us from the love of Christ? Shall trouble or hardship or persecution or famine or nakedness or danger or sword? For I am convinced that neither death nor life, neither angels nor demons, neither the present nor the future, nor any powers, neither height nor depth, nor anything else in all creation, will be able to separate us from the love of God that is in Christ Jesus our Lord. (Rom. 8:35,38–39)

The apostle is telling us that God's love toward us is constant; it is not affected by any outside powers or experiences. God has made us a part of his family, and he never stops loving us. Incomprehensible? Yes, if we judge it by human standards. It is a love that differs from love among humans in that it doesn't vary in accord with our behavior. Although we may sin in the most despicable way, God still loves us. That makes his love unique. It goes beyond all notions of loving someone who loves in return.

As we rejoice in that fact we go beyond the intellect of acquiring information and begin experiencing love emotionally. That is important because love is also an emotional experience. It is experiential. As this happens, the stage is set for true growth in love toward God. It makes us grateful, even awestruck, and it spurs us on to want to know him more intimately, to know his nature. Such was Moses' experience as he talked to God about leading the Israelites:

> If you are pleased with me, teach me your ways, *so I may know you* and continue to find favor with you. (emphasis mine) (Ex. 33:13)

Love and Obedience

How do we get to know his ways? The obvious answer is to look to the Bible, the written revelation that records them. Through that process we are to learn that God views obedience as an integral part of love. That seems a bit harsh because it runs contrary to our concept of loving. We like love to emanate from desire, not from orders. But obedience makes sense when we understand it to be enveloped in love. The two are interrelated, because when we love someone we do everything possible to please and fulfill the desires of that person. That seems to be what Jesus was saying when he taught his disciples about love—that they will express their love toward him by obeying his commands (John 14:15).

But let's not get the wrong idea about this. Loving him is to be a joy, not a burden (I John 5:3). Jesus was not being self-centered. He spoke of loving him for *our* benefit, because his teaching was for *our* well-being. God is always concerned about *us*. That was the essence of God's instructions to Israel of old:

> And now, O Israel, what does the Lord your God ask of you but to fear the Lord your God, to walk in all his ways, to love him, to serve the Lord your God with all your heart and with all your soul, and to observe the Lord's commands and decrees that I am giving you today *for your own good?* (emphasis mine) (Deut. 10:12–13)

That does not ignore God's holiness and the fact that our sins interrupt fellowship with a holy Father. Yes, he is affected by our sins simply because sin is contrary to his divine nature. But he is always concerned about *our* welfare.

Perhaps we can get an inkling of his sorrow over our wrongdoing by thinking about the effect of children's disobedience on their parents. Mothers and fathers can become emotionally wrought over negative behaviors of their offspring. God likewise exhibits emotion, as seen in the Holy Spirit grieving over our sins (Eph. 4:30–32). Without doubt that sorrow stems from his compassion for our well-being. That tenderness is likewise reflected as God sees people's confusion and misdirection in life.

> When he saw the crowds, he had compassion on them, because they were harassed and helpless, like sheep without a shepherd. (Matt. 9:36)

Since God is holy, he yearns for us to be holy, not identical to him of course, for that would be impossible of humans plagued with an inherent sinful nature. But he would have us realize holiness first of all by the act of believing in his Son, which in God's eyes is a holiness (sanctification) that merits eternal life, and then by growing in godliness out of reverence to a merciful heavenly Father (2 Cor. 7:1). It all leads to sweet ongoing fellowship with him.

Spending Time with God

In order to grow in love toward God we must get to know him. The prophet Jeremiah had it right when he said,

> This is what the Lord says: Let not the wise man boast of his wisdom or the strong man boast of his strength or the rich man boast of his riches, but let him who boasts boast about this: that he understands and knows me. (9:23–24)

Knowing God. It is far greater than wisdom, strength and riches. The big question is, how do we know him?

The initial step, of course, is to know him as Savior. But let's go beyond that experience, as crucial as it is. We begin to understand the complexities of a love relationship when we think about the development of human ties. We love our earthly parents because we have developed an intimacy with them through years of close association. Then we marry and grow in love for our spouses. The same can be said about love for our children. I am sure you agree that love doesn't develop without closely shared lives. Conversely, when little time is spent together, love suffers. And when that happens between family members, it opens the door for discord and disaster.

What do you suppose happens to our lives spiritually when we fail to spend time with God? The question looms important given the fact that as spiritual sons and daughters we are declared to be in a family relationship with God (and with one another, by the way). And a family relationship, be it physical or spiritual, isn't merely a product of birth or marriage. It begins there, of course, in both the physical and the spiritual, just as Jesus spoke to Nicodemus about a new birth (John 3:3–7). But a relationship must develop toward intimacy in order for it to remain healthy.

An important key to developing a close relationship with anyone is *communication*. Experts on human relations have been telling us that for years. So it is with our relationship with God, which both the New and Old Testaments have been propagating for several thousand years. Those records of God and man communicating show us the overwhelming importance of communication with God.

Listening to God

The basic spiritual lesson to be learned about hearing God is to recognize his provision of the Bible as his basic means of speaking to us. That may seem stuffy in comparison with hearing God through more spectacular means. But listening to the Bible in large measure represents listening to God. And why would it not be so? After inspiring men to write his critical message about initiating and sustaining a relationship with him, he preserved the writings throughout the ages for all generations to read. That is the Bible we have today. It is a trustworthy document, filled with predictions written hundreds of years prior to their actual fulfillment—prophecies about the Messiah to come, and many other events that took place after they had been predicted. Especially noteworthy in terms of New Testament fulfillment is that which fulfilled Jesus' promise of God indwelling us through the Holy Spirit. That happening, of course, is not convincing to those who don't know him. How could it be? They haven't experienced his indwelling. But for us,

God's personalizing himself is real. Scripture expresses it this way:

> The Spirit himself testifies with our spirit that we are God's children. (Rom. 8:16)

Another biblical passage differentiates between believers and nonbelievers in terms of understanding things God has given us.

> We have not received the spirit of the world, but the Spirit who is from God, that we may understand what God has freely given us. (1 Cor. 2:12)

> The man without the Spirit, does not accept the things that come from the Spirit of God, for they are foolishness to him, and he cannot understand them, because they are spiritually discerned. (v. 14)

These are words we Christians acknowledge as true, because we have experienced their touch in our lives while at the same time see their rejection by the world.

Some have called the Bible "God's love letter" to us. And rightly so, for it tells how he cares for us, wants a personal relationship with us, and ultimately will take us to heaven to enjoy an eternity with him. So there it is—his Holy Word—awaiting us to open its pages and reap its benefits.

There will be some effort involved. At first that requirement may not sound very appealing. We don't like to take the time from our busyness to get familiar with the Bible. It seems like such a big book. We like quick fixes. "Lord, show me what you want of me," we say. But we aren't willing to pay the cost. We want him to zap us in some miraculous way, which means we put the burden on him while we just sit back and wait for the zapping to happen. Which is never.

God has already spoken to us. He has shown us his will in writing. We start the process of learning his will by getting familiar with its content. That written declaration lays out ways of developing a love relationship with the Almighty, some of which we have already seen in our discussion on grace and faith. We will see yet others as we read on. A love relationship is what God wants; it is the way we get to know him and the way he tells us what he wants of us. Look at the emphasis Jesus gave it:

> Love the Lord your God with all your heart and with all your soul and with all your mind. This is the first and greatest commandment. (Matt. 22:37–38)

Mark's gospel adds another phrase to those words of Jesus: that you love God "with all your strength" (Mark 12:30). That translates to loving God with intensity, with one's total being. I don't believe we grasp the entire significance of it automatically, because growing in love is a process. It takes time; we can't seem to absorb God's tenderness all at once. Our love relationship grows as we listen to him communicating at various stages of our lives.

Spending time reading, studying, meditating on God's Word, and even memorizing portions of it, are a help in the listening process. Numerous aids exist through Christian organizations and publishing houses to facilitate it; however, we can accumulate a plethora of such materials and find little benefit if we use them infrequently. Even without that material, that is to say, relying on the Bible alone, we profit little without self-discipline in reading it. The exigencies of life tend to get in the way and must be dealt with through a disciplined approach if we want to grow in love for God through the Scripture. When we want something bad enough, we take steps to see that we get it.

The psalmist in Psalm 119 portrays this kind of attitude toward Scripture. He tells how it helps us:

1. keeping our lives pure (vv. 9–11) (v. 133);
2. strengthening us in times of sorrow (v. 28);
3. giving stability when we are taunted (v. 42);
4. comforting (v. 52);
5. giving wisdom (vv. 98–99) (v. 104);
6. conquering troubles and distress (v. 143);
7. providing peace (v. 165).

That is a wonderful list of benefits. Do you want them? They come through the Bible. The psalmist sees them obtainable as he compares them to a treasure beyond appraisal:

> The law of your mouth is more precious to me than thousands of pieces of silver and gold. (v. 72)

Indeed, as we think about its riches, we see Scripture extend into all aspects of life. The treasure is so vast it truly can't be counted.

You may be currently undergoing one or more of the seven needs listed above. Look at them again, one by one. How do they apply to your life at the moment? One of God's means of helping is through the pages of the Bible. It is one of our greatest sources of strength.

Christians, then, have a provision at their disposal for listening to God, which is like a treasure chest from which we extract riches needed for daily living, indeed for our survival at times. It is God's primary provision for talking to us. Its treasures are there for digging into and scooping up to enrich our lives. The Bible equips us to triumph over all of life's happenings.

The trouble is we want intimacy with God through more spectacular means. Reading the Bible seems an awfully dry experience. Well, we will experience more once we get into the Scriptures. Those sacred pages call attention to God's intimate ways of which we weren't aware, and then we can begin experiencing them.

How do we approach the task of scooping up those biblical treasures? Certainly we aren't going to do an in-depth study of some aspect of the Bible every day. Even professional theologians don't do that. But when our objective is to listen to his communication we will find daily reading to serve us well. In fact, many will attest to the fact that God has a miraculous way of speaking through a Bible passage so as to meet a particular urgency they are facing at the moment.

To maximize benefits from reading the Bible, we will find an added step to be helpful—meditation. I am not talking about a mysterious process associated with non-Christian religions. Rather, I am referring to pondering or thinking about what we read in Scripture. Let's explore what mediation can do for us.

Meditation

Meditating, or thinking about the reading content, helps us scrutinize God's message for personal application. It amounts to digesting what we read, and in the process it allows God to address us intimately through his Spirit on matters he wants to call to our attention. A quickly read biblical passage is prone to be forgotten almost as soon as it is read. Pondering on that passage, however, can give us the joy of a deeper communion with our Lord, one that impacts on our minds for remembrance even beyond that particular day. That is because we often associate our reading with some particular event or experience in our past lives, which then impacts on us by drawing us closer to God.

Scripture tells us of a number of subjects easily associated with meditation. We see the psalmist pondering many of them: God's unfailing love (48:9), his wonders (119:27), decrees (119:48), precepts (119:78), statutes (119:99), promises (119:148), and all his wonderful works (143:5). That covers a lot of territory, but it is not all inclusive. Content will vary for each individual as the Spirit connects and speaks according to our own needs, personalities and background.

Meditation need not be restricted to Bible reading. It can take place in any venue, as in nature, for example, where we may not even have a Bible with us. We can become awestruck over a high mountain range, a trickling stream in the forest, a sandy sea shore, a tumultuous ocean, a waving wheat field, a flower garden bursting with color, a brilliant and splendorous rainbow, or the great expanse of the heavens seen through a starry sky. But meditation is a spiritual force only when the subject matter is associated with God. That is supported by Scripture, as can be seen in some of the psalmist's thoughts:

> O Lord my God, you are very great; you are clothed with splendor and majesty. He wraps himself in light as with a garment; he stretches out the heavens like a tent and lays the beams of his upper chambers on their waters. He makes the clouds his chariot and rides on the wings of the wind. (Ps. 104:1–3)

We may not be as poetic as the psalmist in expressing God's splendor and majesty. Nor should we try. Let each with his own imagination, some more vivid than others, find joy in exulting in God and his handiwork.

That was my experience in South Korea. I was in the city of Pusan to advise on establishing a program in English as a Foreign Language at one of its universities. My hosts, the university president and his deans, suggested taking me to the mountains for a day's outing. Part of that experience was to visit a forest of overwhelming beauty and serenity. Buddhist monks, I was told, often frequented it for meditation.

As I sat there, totally apart from the hustle and bustle of the outside world, I could understand why people would want to go there—to get alone, to absorb the quietness, to think. My focus was almost immediately transferred from self to that of the Creator and his handiwork—the splashes of sun peeking through dense tree tops, a soft wind rustling through the leaves, and the tinkling brook sending its musical sounds ever so lightly in the background. Everywhere was the whisper of the Almighty's presence. "Lord, how great you are," I said. "Thank you for reminding me of your majesty." So real was the Lord's presence that it stayed with me for the rest of my Korean stay. I then carried it home to compose a melody accompanied by the following lyrics:

> Lord, I glorify thy name. Thou, who o'er creation reigns.
> Great thou art. Great thou art, my Lord.
> Oh wonderful, the great I Am, Almighty God.
> Thy majesty, o'erwhelms my soul, commands my heart.
> Lord, I glorify thy name. Thou, who o'er creation reigns.
> Great thou art. Great thou art, my Lord.
> Thy majesty, o'erwhelms my soul, commands my heart.

It represented my response to my Lord for his greatness I had experienced in that Korean forest. And then I was hit by the thought that this great God who created all that beauty has a personal interest in me. It is not an unusual extension of our dwelling on God's majesty.

Meditation, be it inspired by the Bible, by nature, or by whatever, need not be an activity ending in itself. It can wield such an effect on our emotions as to lead to giving thanks and praise. That aspect of prayer, by the way, is something we tend to do very little of in our communication with God. We tend to be "give me" oriented, always asking for favors. Is that what a relationship is all about, asking for things? We would get nowhere doing that with humans. So, with God, why not put aside requests in order to cry out our inner feelings of praise and thanksgiving that result from emotion-laden thoughts? It is showing gratitude. Everybody, including God, likes to hear words of thanks (Ps. 100).

Meditation is a means whereby God calls wonderful things to our attention. It is natural that we talk to him in return. I am suggesting, then, that prayer is a normal extension of meditation. I will have more to say about it under the heading "Talking to God."

Showing Resolve

I would be remiss not to recognize that other activities demanded of us in life, such as working to earn a living, can dominate our lives at the expense of reflecting on God's greatness and love. Of course we have to support ourselves financially, but we don't have to let it control us to the extent of robbing us from listening to God. To allow such to happen is a recipe for defeat, or at least a ho-hum spiritual existence. It applies to the spiritual dimension as well as to the physical realm. By spending little time with the one toward whom you want to grow in love, you end up a loser. That is the way you can lose your spouse or your children.

With God, of course, our relationship in terms of salvation is never severed by our inaction, but we forfeit *the joy of intimacy with him* by failing to grow in love.

Your agreement with this idea of intimacy will be shown by your actions. Just as you would attend to spending more time with your family, so you must do with God. Your family members will see your sincerity as they observe your attention to them. So it is with God. However, our newborn enthusiasm for spending time with God must not end with a mere day or two of renewal and then with a return to old ways. We must make a commitment and keep it! Otherwise Satan seizes upon our inconstancy by causing guilt over our lack of discipline and self-control. But are you aware that in his cunning he will also attack us in the opposite direction—through our resolve for self-discipline? How can that be?

Problems in Self-Discipline

In our challenge to spend time with God by listening to his written revelation we see the importance of self-discipline. It combats life's ongoing demands that rob us of the needed communication. But there is a danger in this process. We can become so consumed by it that we lose sight of its very purpose. It can become an end in itself rather than a means to an end. Without realizing it, we can practice discipline in reading the Bible and find ourselves merely acquiring knowledge. That can cause us to lose sight of the full spiritual benefits it is intended to produce—growth in love toward God.

We can engage in memorizing Scripture, only to find the same thing happening, although perhaps more subtly. It can be connected to selfish ambition, such as to show off our knowledge by quoting verses in front of people, and with their exact references (book, chapter and verse) on top of it. We may even get upset with folks who criticize us as ultra-regimented. "Don't they realize the importance of God's Word in their lives?" we ask. To make them see the folly of their ways we cite Scripture such as: 1 Peter. 2:2–3, Acts 20:32, 2 Timothy 2:15, and 3:16–17, Proverbs 2:6, and Psalm 119, all of which carry the important message of the value of studying and memorizing God's Word.

That was a picture of me in my early years as a Christian. I memorized hundreds of verses followed periodically with an elaborate review system based on daily, weekly, monthly, bimonthly, and semiannual review depending on the newness of the verses memorized. I became obsessed with the process, and I felt proud about it. I actually believed my efforts gave me a corner on truth about knowing God. With that belief came a certain arrogance, kind of like that of the Pharisees and Sadducees of Jesus' day. Acquiring knowledge for ready use before others became my incentive for learning those verses. Yes, it made me appear scholarly, but at the expense of developing intimacy with my Lord. Of course I said I wanted a close relationship with him, but knowledge somehow crowded it out and became the greater focus. It is an example of letting a good principle—listening to God through the Bible—lose its effect on our love relationship with him.

I still believe in scripture memory. Used properly, it enhances love for God, provides ammunition against Satan's attacks of temptation, and facilitates ministering to others. Regarding the latter, however, we must be aware that, like any other spiritual activity, it can produce pride rather than the desired goal of helping others in love. A case in point is a Bible study group in which one of its members announced a vague remembrance of a scriptural passage related to the discussion. As a scripture memory buff I wowed the group by jumping in to quote the exact words and reference of the passage. The group was amazed. My ego soared.

It doesn't have to be that way, of course. But that was often my reaction. And on top of it I pushed scripture memory on others as a means of underscoring one's seriousness about knowing God's Word.

Little did I realize that in my exuberance for knowing the Bible through the process of memorization I was assuming an attitude similar to that of the legalists, those joy-killers I referred to in earlier chapters. The only difference was that I was saying, "*Do* such- and- such," while they were saying "*Don't do* such- and- such." I was so eager for others to follow my example of a disciplined life in the Bible that I became impatient toward them and even critical.

I hope this confession doesn't cause you to downgrade the importance of spending time in the Scripture. I have run the risk of showing you how I abused the use of God's Word. Please receive it as an avoidance procedure rather than as a detractor from the Bible.

Some imagery might be helpful in underscoring the value of Scripture, and even of memorizing it. It is depicted in several ways, some of which are:

> a treasure chest replete with spiritual riches (Ps. 119:72,162); a lamp to light our path (Ps. 119:105); a taste of God sweeter than honey (Ps. 119:103); a seed planted in us that blossoms (Luke 8:11–15); a refuge and shield (Ps. 119:114); food for spiritual nourishment (Matt. 4:4); (1 Peter 2:2); a sword that penetrates one's inner being (Heb. 4:12).

Did you catch the imagery?—a treasure, a lamp, a sweet and pleasant taste, a productive seed, protection, food for growth, and a means of cutting into the thoughts and attitudes of our hearts. In other words, the Bible contains a multiplicity of benefits to enrich our lives. Appropriating those benefits, I started growing in personal awareness of God's marvelous desire for intimacy with me.

There are yet other ways to listen to God. They don't annul the first, the Bible, but rather complement it to enhance our love relationship. Let's read on to see what they are.

Other Communicative Ways

If we are to listen to God we must examine avenues other than the Bible as the means for God to communicate. He does speak apart from Scripture, but we are often insensitive to it. The problem is that people make claims that boggle the mind: dreams, visions, angelic appearances, feelings, mental impressions, audible voices, needs fulfilled, and more. We view many of these experiences as bizarre and unbelievable. Some people reject all of them outright.

Talking about these things runs the risk of turning readers off. But I am going to take that risk on a couple of them. I hope you will consider them with an open mind. By that I mean that you temporarily put aside previous judgments about divine communication and consider the possibility that it exists today in different forms.

I have found that many Christians express reservations about God communicating apart from the Bible. Yet many of them at the same time nod in agreement as they listen to missionaries testifying of divine direction about going to the mission field. Canceling out those directions as invalid would be saying that a vast number of missionary callings are illusion.

How does God communicate intimately apart from the Bible? His primary means, as I see it, is through mental impressions, many of which are confirmed through the Bible as well as through other experiences. They are given when we face momentous events, such as feeling a call to the mission field. But they also pertain to little things of ordinary living. This latter category tends to create misgivings because it allows for excesses that often prove to be nothing more than misguided thinking. However, a balanced view is needed. Yes, some people go off the deep end with crazy thoughts they attribute to God. But it seems to me absurd to dismiss all our thoughts as something of our own doing. God the Father, Son and Holy Spirit consider believers in Christ as special, and therefore the Divine has put himself within us to counsel us (John 14:16–17, 23, 25). Our role is to be judicious listeners so as to not make a mockery of that privileged process.

When I raise the subject of God's communication on everyday happenings, I often get blank stares. People tell me they have never experienced such a phenomenon. It is not that God doesn't communicate with them on little things of ordinary living. They just haven't been conscious of it, and therefore the communication goes unrecognized. When that happens, don't expect God to beat you over the head and tell you to wake up. He is gentle. He will keep trying to get through to you in other situations. It will all be for your growth in love for him—the enjoyment of Christianity to the fullest.

In my early years as a Christian I didn't have the slightest clue of God's communication apart from the Bible. No one ever sat down to explain it to me. Neither were there people around me whose lives I could use as examples. I knew that the Bible spoke of the Holy Spirit living within me and serving to direct my paths, but I interpreted it solely as God's means of telling me to avoid sin. After all, the Spirit is grieved when we do bad things, the Bible says (Eph. 4:30–32). I had to learn that God communicates beyond reminders of bad behavior.

Later in my Christian experience, people kept telling me that God spoke to them in all kinds of situations of personal significance. However, I thought it quite absurd, since I knew how imagination can run wild. But the more I observed the lives of those claiming this intimate touch, the more I began to consider its credibility. They weren't like me—nervous, distraught, and straining to be in control. Rather, they exhibited a peacefulness, a rest, and a relinquishing of self-effort that seemed so attractive. I wanted it. It signaled an important step in enjoying the fruits of a love relationship with Christ.

If I am to believe that God is an intimate Father who desires fellowship with me, then that must mean more than his restraining influence on bad behavior. So I decided to sit back, pay attention to my thoughts, and then consider the possibility of those thoughts being God sent.

They were messages about little things, items of significance only to me. You may be saying, "How about some examples?" Well, okay. It is a question I also asked as I read books about intimacy with God whose authors gave no personal examples. I often wondered whether those writers really knew from experience what they were talking about.

Most recent and fresh in memory over the past few weeks are three different communications: comfort after being snubbed; reminder of the blessing of finances; and, confirmation about returning to the classroom to teach part-time. I will explain these impressions below. But first, I have to confess that I hesitated to list any examples at all out of fear they would seem trivial or meaningless to someone else. Worse yet, I feared you might think me a candidate for the funny farm. "He hears voices," you might say.

Audible messages? Absolutely not! If that were so, I don't think I could handle it. I know myself. Pride would start popping up about favoritism with God, as if I were in a class with Abraham, Moses, Paul, or some other personality to whom God spoke orally. Or I might not even accept the validity of the message, because I am good at rationalizing things away. "I didn't really hear anything," I might say. "It was just my imagination." That is why I don't expect to actually hear God's audible voice. I am just not good material for him in that respect. And I suspect that is true for most of us, especially for us professors. We are so analytical.

But let's get back to the nonverbal messages. You deserve that I explain them. That inclusion here is in itself a step of faith on my part. Although the detail may not be meaningful to everyone, it may be just what someone needs for seeing God's communicative process more clearly at work in his or her own life.

1. **Snubbed.** Snubbed means I was overlooked and my feelings crushed. I was bypassed in handling a teaching activity at my church, which caused me discouragement, hurt, and maybe even a touch of resentment. I had done nothing wrong to warrant being ignored. In fact, I had submitted a proposal for a program under consideration that required considerable labor on my part, one that would have been acted upon immediately by other churches. God knew my disappointment and came to my rescue saying, "I understand. But your timing is not right. Patience! I am with you. Remember, I know all things." I believed, I rested, and I had peace.
2. **Finances.** Within one week three fellow believers shared their concerns with me about their dwindling finances. A significant reduction of income was producing serious hardship for them. I of course made it a special part of my intercessory prayer, and I even

offered to contribute financially to meeting their needs. At the same time, however, I had the urge to give God praise and thanks for *my* steady income—a reminder of a divine blessing from a generous heavenly Father. I realized my need to render greater acknowledgment of God's blessings and not to take them for granted. God was reminding me of his care. God is good. I felt compelled to tell him so.

3. **Teaching.** For some time my thoughts were directed to a return to the classroom as an adjunct (part-time) professor. I had been undergoing a period of inactivity as a retiree that was beginning to get me down. I felt that the academic environment would be stimulating through its provision for intellectual interaction with faculty colleagues. And who knows? Maybe it would open doors for a ministry with students, I thought. Would one of the area colleges be interested in my services, I wondered? I wasn't sure what their attitude would be toward a retiree. After sending out feelers and waiting three months for a response, I received a phone call announcing that a course had just become available. Would I be interested? they asked.

So why am I crediting God for all of this? Because I felt that he instilled in me the thought to pursue re-entry to the academic scene in the first place. And just as I accepted it on faith, so with faith I anticipate results God will cause to happen in me and perhaps through me with colleagues and students. It is called closeness with God based on a very personal and intimate love relationship.

You will notice that each communication is of a different kind. One deals with comfort, while another with praise. Unlike the teaching position, the veracity of those two encounters can't be confirmed by hard evidence seen in a future happening. You could argue that they were products of my own thoughts. But I don't accept them that way, mainly because I know my personality. It doesn't generally cause me to think about accepting comfort and giving thanks for finances. I am learning the beauty of those characteristics. But essentially you are hearing from a strong man, one raised to be self-reliant. So, to what do I attribute those messages? The only answer I have is, to God.

God's communication is sometimes confirmed through events that happen in the future, such as my return to the classroom. At other times it coincides with biblical content, such as being forgiving and patient, praising him for his goodness, and contributing to the needs of the saints. Yet at other times I simply accept God's communication through whatever means he chooses to use. I see it all as an expression of his love and his desire that I grow in love for him.

I recall a few strains of an old hymn I used to sing in college. It expresses nicely my sentiment about friendship with Jesus.

> There's not a friend like the lowly Jesus. No, not one!
> No, not one!
>
> There's not an hour that he is not near us. No, not one!
> No, not one!

That nearness spells intimate friendship with Jesus—an ingredient of communication.

I now am going to take a big risk to talk about another of God's means of speaking. I classify it as an extraordinary event because it is so infrequent. In fact, it may well be a one-in-a million event. Yet my experience with it tells me of its veracity. What is it? God's angelic messengers! Whoa!

you may say. That happened in Bible times, but not now. I hope you will read my account with an open mind, all to the end of seeing God communicating love to his children in very trying circumstances. My experience is tied to that last phrase—very trying circumstances. I think that as you hear my story you will understand why I put credence in extraordinary acts of communication. But above all, please keep the end result in mind—that God communicates in very special circumstances to remind his children of his love. Concentrating on the means, the miraculous event alone, will detract from seeing the end result of God's tender expression of love.

I emphasize at the outset that the appearance of angels is not a usual happening. Far be it for me to suggest that it will happen to you. The message I want to send, however, is that God may use such an event to meet a severe, drastic need in someone's life. Not everyone experiences such hardships. But when they do, they may be the recipients of God's love in unusual ways. That is my purpose in relating this story—God loves us.

In spite of the fact that angelic appearances are mentioned frequently in the Bible, I can cite only one instance of it in my lifetime. And then the bizarre event was not one of my own experience but that of my late wife, Kay, who received that divine communication and blessing prior to her death. It was a breathtaking event for me when I learned of it. It shattered all my logic on God's ways of communicating to us today. Here is what happened.

In one of my daily visits to the nursing home during Kay's last months of life, I told her about a television program I had seen the night before that presented accounts of angelic appearances in the lives of several people. Taken back by some of the reports connecting angels to cosmic spirits with no reference to God or Jesus Christ, I related the program with some degree of skepticism and even derision. To my astonishment she began groaning, obviously reflecting displeasure with my attitude. She was telling me in no uncertain terms to stop criticizing. "What do you mean?" I asked. "Are you trying to tell me you agree with the idea of angelic appearances today? Are you telling me you've seen an angel?" I was hoping it wasn't so. A husband, sensitive to his wife's suffering hardly wanted to upset an already distraught woman with his reaction of unbelief.

Probing with this dear woman whose speech had deteriorated almost to the point of extinction, I pursued the matter with a series of yes/no questions, which took considerable time, since that kind of inquiry required thinking of every possible angle to get the detail of the account. Questioning even had to extend to the next day because of its fatigue on Kay. We followed our usual communicative process—a squeeze of my hand when she wanted to reply in the affirmative. Here is what I learned.

In the middle of the night, when Kay was experiencing a horrid time of pain and sadness, a woman dressed in ordinary street clothes (we can rule out the nurses, who wear uniforms) stood at the foot of her bed. She spoke, remained there smiling for a minute or so, and then exited the room. "What did she say?" I eagerly but stupidly asked, forgetting for the moment that Kay's speech difficulty made it impossible for her to talk. To my astonishment, she managed with a faint voice to answer my query with two whispered words: "Be Happy!" My immediate reaction was one of anger, extreme anger. Be happy? "What kind of message is that?" I said to myself. "My wife is dying, and she's supposed to be happy?" I suspect she noted my agitation because, in a whisper of barely audible tones, she forced out five more words, five remarkable words—"He takes care of me." That utterance would have been lost to my ears had I not been perceptive enough to watch Kay's lip movements. It had been a long time since she had vocalized, albeit softly, to such an extent.

Overcome with wonder as to what this all meant, I sat in silence pondering the experience. (I've often wondered since then what Kay was thinking as I sat there with a dumbfounded look on my face.) Finally, it dawned on me that God might be preparing to take her to himself, to have her leave behind her tortured existence for a marvelous new life in heaven . . . a place where she would be free of pain, crying, and sadness. Why not give her a message to "Be Happy?" It made sense. Shortly thereafter, that new life became reality for her.

This amazing experience convinced this skeptical, academically oriented husband that God does indeed speak to his children in unusual ways. After 10 long years of suffering with her disease, Kay needed that communication. And God knew it. It underscored for me that the divine personal message filled her very urgent need for assurance and comfort. It must have increased her faith and love for her Creator even more. God's words, "Be Happy!" along with Kay's response, "He takes care of me," were Kay's last spoken words to me. They of course burned an indelible mark on my mind. They are words all of us might carry with us as a reminder of God's presence in whatever circumstances we may encounter.

For Kay, the experience was unquestionably one causing an array of mixed feelings. She wanted release from her tortured existence, yet at the same time she undoubtedly sorrowed over having to leave husband, children and grandchildren. Happy memories of loved ones probably always make approaching death difficult. But I wonder if at that austere moment she was not thinking of Chapter Two of the Song of Songs, which in earlier days I had put to music. Kay used to go about singing the key strains:

> O my beloved he comes, he speaks and says to me,
> Arise my love, my fair one, and come away with me.
>
> For lo the winter is past, the rains are over and gone,
> Flowers appear on the earth, the time of singing has come.
>
> Arise, my love, my fair one, and come away with me.
>
> Arise, my love, my fair one, and come away with me.

Obviously they would have been appropriate words for Kay to remember in her final days.

Her angel experience is certainly not unique. Others have reported the involvement of divine beings in their lives. Verification of those accounts is impossible, but for those who experience them, none is needed. We do have, however, the sure word of Scripture that tells us that angels are among us. The book of Hebrews talks about them.

> Are not all angels ministering spirits sent to serve those who will inherit salvation? (Heb. 1:14)

And also,

> Do not forget to entertain strangers, for by so doing some people have entertained angels without knowing it. (Heb. 13:2)

Of course biblical examples of angelic appearances abound, some of which are: with Moses at the burning bush; with Hagar, mother of Ishmael; with Abraham and the destruction of Sodom and Gomorrah, and also prior to his preparation to sacrifice Isaac; and, with Jacob prior to meeting his brother Esau. Numerous situations likewise are recorded in the New Testament, some of which are: the angelic announcement to the virgin Mary of her miraculous pregnancy; the appearance to the women at Jesus' empty tomb; the angel coming to Peter in prison; and, the angel allaying Paul's fear for his life in the stormy sea.

Angels sent by God to help his children. It isn't a common happening, to be sure, but one that God may choose at times to communicate with us. It all fits under our topic of listening to God—God telling us something very special in desperate circumstances.

I have never personally experienced a supernatural appearance of God's heavenly messengers, and I suspect most others have not either. But I have learned not to limit God. He is the Sovereign Most High who can create whatever means he wishes to communicate with us. When he does, its meaningfulness of course is personally convincing. The problem that may arise, however, is that in our enthusiasm we go off the deep end and start proclaiming God's supernatural communication as normative for all Christians. I have come to acknowledge that God indeed uses unusual forms to reveal himself at times, but he seems to do so only when we are in special need of help. He comes to our rescue, but only he decides how, when, where, and if it is to be done.

There is something, however, that distresses me about talk of extraordinary divine communication. Some people speak of it as if it were an ongoing occurrence involving trivial matters. Their speech is so loaded with what I call "God told me's" that they sound like Old Testament prophets. So let's see what that is all about.

God Told Me

I know Christians who continually talk about God giving them messages. It is a kind of super spiritual talk I suspect they use as a device to lend authority to what they say. I suppose people who speak that way feel that their message is more likely to be received if they associate it with "heavenly origin." To make matters worse, they seldom, if ever, explain this "God-told-me-business" in terms of how it was given. In most instances listeners don't usually ask, maybe out of fear of being perceived as nonspiritual or even argumentative, or in their kindness they may simply not want to put the speaker on the spot.

No, I am not contradicting myself about God speaking to us. I am not talking about those frequent even daily whispers of God's love, direction, and even correction that underscore our intimate walk with him. We thrive spiritually on such personalized communication. What I am saying is, "Watch out that you don't declare your imagination as God-given communication."

God does indeed talk to us, but when he does so apart from the Bible, a safe approach is to evaluate it in terms of its consistency with Scripture. If there is a contradiction we can be sure the message is not of God. For example, two people in love, try to justify premarital sex because they feel God has told them it is okay now that they have promised themselves to each other for marriage. Strong personal desires such as sexual impulses have their way of controlling thought processes to the extent of rationalizing away God-given principles (in this case, scriptural teaching against sex before marriage) (1 Cor. 6:13–18; 7:2) (Eph. 5:3) (1 Thess. 4:3–4). Clergymen with liberal leanings toward interpretation of Scripture may condone premarital sex (more politely described today as "living together"), or at least look the other way when they suspect church members who engage in it. They defend their attitude as one of kindness and love as they assent to premarital sex for an engaged couple, reasoning that in God's eyes they are already married spiritually on the basis of their promise to each other. The counseled ones like that kind of logic; it is what they want to hear. It sounds so humane, so understanding. And it must be okay with God, they conclude. "After all, his minister condones it." Ouch!

This is not the place to explore the topic of sexual immorality. I cite the above as but an example of how we can believe we have received a message from God, even though it contradicts Scripture, and for that matter, in this case, society's legal definition of marriage. Why, the couple even had confirmation through the pastor that their premarital sex message had to be God-given. We must be careful to differentiate between our own emotions and divine communication.

Another consideration relative to belief in God's communication has to do with highly personal circumstances that the Bible doesn't address. For example, we might have an urgent feeling to call on a friend. We wonder if it is of God. Oftentimes the immediate outcome, such as finding that person desperately in need of help, verifies the divine nature of the communication. Recognizing that our minds can deceive us, however, it seems best to declare the "God told me" message *after* the communication is substantiated as God-given, not *before*. This has nothing to do with lack of faith; rather it recognizes our vulnerability to error in regard to mental activity.

A case in point is the story of my friend Bill (not his real name), who dismissed God's wisdom as proclaimed in the Bible by marrying an unbeliever. He soon experienced great grief in finding that his wife wanted nothing to do with his spiritual concerns—his church, his Christian friends, the Bible, and Christianity in general. One of the ladies of his church, having observed Bill's sadness over the matter, assured him that everything would turn out all right, because God had *told her* that Bill's wife would ultimately become a believer. That was 35 years ago. His wife is just as antagonistic as ever. And Bill's sorrow has increased over that time span, as life with an unbelieving spouse bitterly unfolded for him: attending church alone; entertaining Christian friends in his home while an intolerant wife refused to participate; and, perhaps most heartbreaking of all, seeing his children grow up rejecting Christianity out of influence of their mother.

It is a heart-wrenching story, but not to overshadow my purpose in telling it. "God told me" can be a dangerous utterance. We must not allow our emotions to dictate in declaring it. A check on that verbal behavior is to ask ourselves, "Are we willing to risk dishonoring God by claiming a future happening that doesn't come to pass?" I have heard evangelists making predictions, and the future proved them wrong. God warned Israel about people who, making themselves to be prophets of God, spoke of future events that never came about (Deut. 18:22). I will be careful in what I call divine communication. No, I don't consider that to be a lack of faith. I consider it judicious, because I know my human vulnerability to emotion.

Out of fear that this discussion may turn you off about God speaking apart from the Bible, I want to remind you that I find God indeed showing intimacy in ways that can't be substantiated by future outcomes. They fall into the category of what I will call "love relationships." It is a theme running throughout this book. Let's not lose sight of personalized divine communication. Only the recipient can substantiate it as God-given, because it is so highly personal. It supports the whole concept behind this writing, that of a continuing personal relationship with God. Such a relationship began at the time of our salvation and receipt of the Holy Spirit, but it is one he wants to develop into a communion of intimacy. That kind of a union is crucial to our joy and well-being. Indeed it is an underlying component of grace, faith, and love which contributes to our spiritual health.

Talking to God

God not only talks to us, he would have us talk to him. Communication is a two-way street, and Jesus encouraged us to engage in it. I have already mentioned the subject in previous pages as I discussed the benefits of meditation. However, there is more to be said.

Talking to God is an urging seen throughout the Bible because it allows for telling him our deepest and most intimate thoughts. And what a marvelous scene it is—sons and daughters coming into the presence of their heavenly Father to speak with him. And, of course, he listens. The Bible declares it.

> For the eyes of the Lord are on the righteous and his ears are attentive to their prayer. (1 Peter 3:12)

Don't let that word "righteous" throw you, as if it means one who is living a perfect and holy life. God declares us righteous when we put our faith in Jesus Christ (Rom. 5:19). It is not a question of living a sinless life, simply because no one can do it.

Although talking to God often involves cries for help, which is an important act in times of distress, it encompasses other communication as well. The psalmist spoke to God in praise, adoration and thanksgiving, in addition to pleas for mercy and intervention. The Christian is urged to do the same, but the meaningfulness of prayer is tied to our intimacy with him. It is unlikely that we will offer up that kind of prayer unless we are abounding in a love relationship.

If our prayers are merely a voicing of our needs, that says something about the limitations of our fellowship. It reveals a restricted and flimsy relationship coming from a selfish desire to fulfill our own wants. On the other hand, as we recognize the abundance of ways in which God is involved in our lives, we have reason to talk to him about matters other than requests.

Physical parents don't want their children to talk with them only when they have needs or when they want something. "Hey, is that all we're good for?" they may ask. "How about telling us about other things . . . maybe your joys and times of discouragement. And while you're at it, it would be nice if you didn't just talk about yourself. Maybe you could voice at times your appreciation of us. We count too, don't we? Hey, we're family."

Ah yes, family. Does that remind us of our relationship with God? So when we approach our heavenly Father as his sons and daughters, what do we talk about? I woke up exceptionally early one morning, sat down in my favorite chair, and thought, "What do I say to my Lord this morning?" My mind raced with all kinds of requests for help, both for myself and for others. Wait a minute. Can't I just talk to God to enjoy him? A whole string of thoughts suddenly appeared for which I could give him praise. I was overwhelmed with the multitude of ideas that came to mind about his interaction with his creation and his provisions for our spiritual and physical well-being. I ended up thanking and praising him for his goodness.

The next time you go to God in prayer, decide to start out talking to him exclusively in terms of thanksgiving and praise. If you are like me, you will find it hard to do at first. You will be amazed how quickly you run out of ideas. You will likely start mixing in petitions so that your prayer time will not be ridiculously short. If you must ask for help, try limiting it to help in praising him. That little exercise will show you how pitifully self-centered our prayers tend to be. We have trouble talking to God *about him*. Our minds tend to revert to talking *about ourselves*. Forget yourself for the moment and concentrate exclusively on him!

Then you can extend your prayers to other matters. I find it helpful to think about the day's events and how he pertains to them. I will undoubtedly recall instances that stir me to give thanks and praise, to adore, to intercede for others, as well as to talk about my own needs. Without this time of reflection, prayer time tends to be difficult. I need times of silence, something that doesn't seem to fit naturally into the busyness of the day. That means I must take steps to provide for that quiet, intimate time with my Lord. Each of us will be different in determining time and place to do that, but we must do it if we are to enjoy the riches of communicating with our heavenly Father.

Of course, a consciousness of God's intervention throughout the day can direct us to talk to God at any moment also. It is being God-conscious in all of our daily experiences—what we do, say, see, hear, and feel. It reflects our intimacy with him each step of the way. That is what Paul may have had in mind when he admonished us to "pray continually" (1 Thess. 5:17). I think that means to acknowledge God's personal involvement throughout the day. It is learning to become communication conscious with him, to give him thanks, praise, adoration and as well as to request his merciful intervention.

One day, for example, I found myself reflecting on several situations about which I wanted to acknowledge God's involvement: a good report from the doctor on my physical condition; developing a relationship with my neighbor; my son landing a long-awaited job; and, my grandchildren performing well in school. So I poured out my heart in thanksgiving. I never thought about doing such a thing in my younger days. I had considered occurrences of this sort as things that just happened to come about. That was so because back then I didn't have the love relationship with God that I am now growing in. I have come to realize that God is involved in every aspect of life, and that he receives my prayers of thanks as a sweet expression of gratitude, or as the writer of Hebrews said, "a sacrifice of praise—the fruit of lips that confess his name" (Heb. 13:15).

I have suggested a number of ways we can enhance communication with God and thus show our love toward him. Biblical admonitions reflect many approaches. References abound on prayer. We are told how, when, where, why, for what, and for whom to pray as well as examples of what Jesus and many others in the Bible prayed about. It is not my purpose to expound on those references. Others have already done a far better job than I could. But I do want to challenge you to think about reflecting your personal love relationship with your Lord as you pray. Does an intimacy exist between you and God? He wants it, and you can have it.

To be fair, I must acknowledge the discouragement many Christians face when they cry out desperately for help and get no immediate answer. I used to be among them, and I still get aggravated about it at times. That is the intellect coming out in me, influencing me to think that I know how God should respond to solve my problems. Yes, I still find myself dictating to God.

We see family and friends suffering horrible diseases, for example, and we lose patience when God fails to come to the rescue. This is where it seems appropriate to pull together the thoughts discussed earlier on grace, faith, and love. Combining these attributes develops in us a spiritual dimension that says, "Lord, I don't understand why you don't heal this malady (or whatever the problem may be), but I know you're in control, and I trust you." Do you remember Paul's "thorn in the flesh" and his reaction to it? That is love—trusting God no matter the outcome.

As we grow older and wiser spiritually we see God's purposes in withholding his power. His will may be to teach us something that he sees good for us to learn, including hardship, but it will all be directed toward bringing us into a greater love relationship with him. Satan tells us this is not reality. "It's nonsense," he shouts. But risking the accusation of being simplistic, we remind ourselves that this God whom we serve is always loving. It is his nature.

Regardless of the position he takes on our petitions, we admit we don't have all the answers. God does. Through faith in that fact we continue in love toward him. It is an important step in dealing with life's happenings . . . loving him no matter what.

A Test of Love

I began this chapter on *Loving God* by suggesting its connection with intimacy, which implies the fallacy that love is mere knowledge. Love is something to be practiced, not just known about. A good test in this regard is to ponder heaven. Why do we want to go there? Have you ever thought about it? It may be instructive to stop reading for a few minutes right now to answer the question, "Why do I want to go to heaven?"

All Christians want to go to heaven, but we give different reasons. We know that Jesus said he was going to prepare a place for us so that we may be there along with him—a promise that involves our eternal destiny, which is why we believed in Christ in the first place.

But then there arises the question of timing. Some people may not want to go to heaven just yet, hoping for a delay because they have material hopes and dreams yet unfulfilled: an impending marriage; the birth of a child; the purchase of a new home; an embarking on an exciting career; or sadness in having to leave family members, such as a spouse, children and grandchildren. Your self-analysis may have included similar thoughts about timing. Such reasons are understandable in the sense that they encompass joyous aspects of life we love to experience. But they quickly fade as we see their temporality, except maybe for the people-oriented ones we find hard to give up because of the human ties involved.

Others may respond to the subject of heaven by by-passing the question. They say they don't really want to think about it until they have lived a full life on earth. In other words, they look to heaven merely as a place to go for continued living beyond the grave. Nothing immediate there.

Then again, an attitude of delay may indicate looking at heaven merely as a means of avoiding hell. After all, who wants an eternity of punishment? We are so consumed with life on earth that we may view heaven merely as an escape route, a kind of using Jesus to avoid the horrors of eternal separation from God. I suspect that many, if not most of us, became Christians for that very reason—to escape punishment for our sins—which is okay, since the gospel message includes that aspect of Jesus' sacrifice for us.

We all want to go to heaven. There is no question about it. But we can't seem to escape setting our own time frame.

But wanting a delay is hardly wrong. It recognizes that our earthly life constitutes the realm of actual experience. It is reality, a life that we know, and for most of us it is enjoyable. We cling to it.

But what about looking upon heaven as a place to go right now, the sooner the better, so to speak? What reasons might be offered? Let's explore.

First, it may be to reunite with family members who have died. That is an understandable motive. After all, some people may have spent most of their earthly lives with spouses who have gone on before. There is great sadness. They miss their mates who have been an integral part of their lives. They have shared joys and sorrows together for many years, if not for most of their lives. Isn't it natural to yearn for reuniting with them? I think so.

Then we must not forget mothers and fathers, and maybe sons or daughters, who have died, memories of whom bring sorrow and tears. It is a natural longing to be with them again.

Another reason for wanting heaven now may be that pain, either physical or mental, reduces the quality of life to such an extent that sufferers want out of this world as quickly as possible. Life for them is hard, and they know that death followed by heaven will be their release. We understand that stance, especially if we are experiencing that very thing right now, or if we have witnessed the intense suffering of a loved one with a fatal disease.

Then there may be another reason, one that smacks of far more importance than any of the others—that of simply wanting to be in Jesus' presence. Did your self-analysis include that notion? If so, I hope it wasn't just "church talk," you learned by being around "spiritual" people. It is also possible that you mechanically support this position with Scripture, like the one about Paul desiring to depart and be with Christ (Phil. 1:23). But could you possibly fail to understand Paul's feelings that led him to say that?

Why did Paul view Jesus as the principal reason for wanting to go to heaven? Through the many passages that express his devotion to Christ we see the great love he had for his Lord. But some may contend that comparing Paul with themselves is unfair. His closeness with the Lord, they suggest, was due to the absence of a love relationship, an intimacy, with someone on earth. After all, they say, his entire life seemed wrapped up with Jesus and his evangelical work for him. It was as if he didn't have a love relationship with anyone else, which would surely point to absence of intimacy and consequent lack of emotional ties with people.

Not so! Although Paul seems to imply that he was not married, at least at the time of his ministry (1 Cor. 9:5), he surely had close relationships with people. The Bible is silent about his parents or other members of his physical family, but it shows his love for those within his spiritual family. Look how he referred to Timothy, for example, his faithful companion in the ministry, whom he tenderly called "my son whom I love" (1 Cor. 4:17).

In spite of closeness with Timothy, and probably with others as well, Paul's earthly relationships apparently took a back seat to his love relationship with Christ. He had developed an intimacy with his Lord that far exceeded any he held with people on earth. Two crucial questions emerge that we can learn from: How did he get such a relationship, so that going to heaven to be with Jesus became his priority; and, what application can there be for my life?

It certainly is not a matter of knowledge of the gospel: that is to say, what I have learned about God's goodness and mercy in saving me. If it were knowledge alone, I might be using Christ merely as a means for life beyond the grave. I think it stems rather on affection, on the level of love I develop with him throughout life that makes the difference.

Since I still cling to selfish desires in wanting heaven, like being with deceased family members, I have to say I am learning about love toward God and intimacy with him to be a growth process, one that requires a great deal of communion together. I suspect that is what Paul was referring to when he spoke of his intense desire to know Christ (Phil. 3:10). I don't pretend to understand all he was thinking in that respect, except that his attitude seemed to be one of complete surrender to living for and with Christ in all of life's activities here on earth (Phil. 1:21).

If I apply that attitude toward another human being, like a spouse, for example, I suppose I am getting pretty close to understanding Paul's attitude. I don't see it as something that comes easily or automatically. We learn from the letter to the Galatians that, following Paul's conversion on the road to Damascus, he spent three years in Arabia which, among other things, was undoubtedly designed to establish intimacy with Christ. Three years of listening to God! I suspect that from then on Paul and God communicated with each other in all circumstances surrounding the apostle's life—stoning, imprisonment, shipwreck, physical ailments, visions, preaching, conversions, and much more. His was a walk of both hardship and joy, but in it all he seemed to grow in love with his Lord by listening attentively to him, and then by serving him.

If we use the marital relationship as an analogy of growth in love, we must acknowledge an important element that makes it work—mutual giving. Love doesn't truly develop when only one of the persons does the giving. It seems fair to say, then, that with love in the spiritual sense, Christians, in addition to expressing love toward God through various means, must experience God's expressions of love toward them. I am not saying that God doesn't do his part. He is constantly working in our lives through a multitude of ways, even as he did for Paul, although I am afraid we often fail to ascribe those happenings to their divine source.

It wasn't until recently that I began to consider God's show of love toward me in my earlier years as a Christian. I recalled blessings for which I had failed to give him credit.

How vivid is the memory, for example, of moving my family from Oklahoma to Georgia and finding a bleak housing market in the university town of Athens. Homes for sale were nonexistent due to a heavy influx of newly hired faculty members who had gotten there months before me. Hunting relentlessly but without success, I finally drove up a street where a man was pounding a For Sale by Owner sign into the ground. His wife had just divorced him, and he wanted out of that house fast. It was a beautiful home, and with five bedrooms to accommodate my large family at that. Just what we needed. But for years I attributed the find to happenstance. What luck, I thought. I can just picture God shaking his head in disbelief over my lack of perception. Yet in all his graciousness he didn't stop loving me. He continued to give, not necessarily in momentous occasions as in finding me a home in a new city, but in the little more frequent happenings of daily life that are personally meaningful.

I have learned to be more attuned to God's goodness as I see his gifts continuing to flow in my direction, although in my human weakness I still fail to recognize them at times, mostly when I foolishly think that when good happens it is because of my own efforts. That is self protruding its ugly head. But aside from these foul-ups, I look back and see God loving me continually, and it spurs me on to love him in return, which gets me one step closer to wanting to be with him in heaven.

So, it is showing love one to another, a love that emanates from both parties, from me and from God, that develops intimacy. But it is my experience that the Lord doesn't wait for me to love him before he does anything. God's actions are characterized by grace, that is, giving without requiring anything in return. He continually showers his blessings on me which, when recognized, spur me on to an intimacy that causes me to yearn falling before him in gratitude for his love.

We cite various reasons for going to heaven. We like the idea of eternal life beyond this world, but many of us would rather not leave our present life just now, simply because it is the only one we know through actual experience. Heaven, on the other hand, albeit a wonderful place, remains mysterious. We know of it only academically. Maybe that is where we go wrong. We think of it as a place, when actually our thoughts ought to be centered around a person—Jesus—with whom we can actually begin a close, experiential relationship on earth.

How do we get this Christ-centered mindset, this love relationship with Jesus? It seems to stem from an intimate walk with him, even as Paul experienced, one which the Bible seems to indicate as something to be greatly desired. But I have found that kind of closeness hardly coming instantly. Even Paul indicated that. We grow in it as we recognize Jesus more as a friend, a dearly beloved spouse, if you will, who yearns for us to recognize his frequent demonstrations of love to each of us personally.

A spousal relationship, by the way, is not foreign to Scripture; it depicts Jesus as the bridegroom and us as his bride. In heaven that relationship will be fully realized when we are present with him at the "Wedding Supper of the Lamb" (Rev. 19:9). I am glad I have been invited. Aren't you? What a joyous time it will be.

It is that intimacy with Jesus that looms as our challenge. The more we grow in it, the more we will likely connect heaven with Jesus. I will relish uniting with loved ones gone on before, and I know I will enjoy the multitude of other delights heaven has to offer. But my focus will be on Jesus, giving him thanks for making it all possible.

In my humanness I continue to cherish earthly ties. Jesus doesn't hold it against me, since he created me and understands human bonds, even as he experienced them while on earth. Yet, it is Jesus, Savior and best friend, who is becoming my focal point . . . the one who merits all my praise, adoration, gratitude and thanksgiving.

Learning to love Jesus. It cuts across all aspects of life, from the time we accepted his generous gift of salvation to thoughts of our demise and spending eternity with him. Love relationships. That is what the Christian life is all about.

But it isn't just a question of developing love for God and stopping there. Love for God finds its natural extension to loving people. That is what God wants, and that is what gives us joy—helping people. We will see in the next chapter some ways that it is done.

CHAPTER 5

Loving Christians

"Serve one another in love."

Galatians 5:13

What constitutes love toward Christians, and how does it take place? Common interrogatives such as what, why, when and where are appropriate to consider in this regard. By doing so we come to better understand personal obligation to love and how to put it into practice. Its effect will cause us to re-evaluate our individual roles as Christians in complying with God's will to love one another, which won't simply be out of mere recognition of a nice sounding concept without taking action to put it into practice. Blessings are to be enjoyed through it, which God intends for each of us to have.

Different Meanings

The English language uses the single word *love* to communicate different aspects of that emotion. We say "love" in expressing a mother's bond with her child, or the binding together of husband and wife, while at the same time we refer to the sexual act as "making love," often referred to as "free love" by those who believe in sexual pleasure without commitment. Regarding the latter, free love, Chesterton viewed it as a misnomer, since he believed that love can't be free. [1] True love requires commitment. I will use that concept as the guiding force for understanding our topic of love in this chapter.

Implications of Commitment

Applying commitment to human relationships, we can say that love is not merely words but deeds. This is what the apostle John wanted us to understand when he said,

> Dear children, let us not love with words or tongue but with actions and in truth. (1 John 3:18)

This is a love that is binding. It is what Chesterton inferred when he spoke of the nature of love—it binds. [2] The logical conclusion is that we must identify with people and then go beyond shallow pronouncements of love which allow for hiding things from one another. The more we avoid that superficiality, the more we will be able to be open with one another and to truly love as reflected in binding people together. Even spouses, by virtue of their intimacy in marriage, fail at times to fully reveal their inner feelings to one another. Such withholding, if habitual, can lead to serious marital problems.

How then can we identify with people beyond superficial relationships? We do it by recognizing that all human beings share a common nature showing itself in feelings of fear, joy, sadness, perplexities, worries, hopes and desires, to identify only a few of the emotions we commonly experience. In short, we want people to empathize with us regarding what we are undergoing. That involves open talk—genuine sharing, without masks to hide our true selves. The trouble is that few of us get close enough to each other to voice our true feelings. Furthermore, we are afraid to do it out of fear that by unmasking we will reveal our faults and then lose the respect of others as they begin to think less of us.

How do Christians get to know each other so as to be able to show mutual care? We do it by getting in an environment where we see spiritual care being given. Where is that? Our quick response is to say, "in church," because that is the logical place where Christians meet and learn about love. "Church," generally interpreted as the Sunday morning worship service, is a good starting place. But I would like to suggest something else we need, another kind of contact for growing in love for one another.

The gathering of several hundred people in the typical one-hour Sunday morning worship service has its limitations. It does not necessarily establish relationships among those attending. We don't even know a lot of the people's names, let alone getting close to one another. And of course it is even worse in the mega churches where thousands gather.

The nature of the Sunday service lends itself pretty much to corporate worship. In fact, it is now called a "worship" service in most churches. Recognizing that people's interaction is an important part of one's spiritual development, churches try to fill that need by including Sunday school classes in their programs. It is a helpful inclusion in giving members greater familiarity with the Bible. However, growth in closeness taking place among adult class members can be minimal due to such factors as revolving attendance, large classes, and the precedence of acquiring Bible knowledge over shared personal application.

This deficiency has caused some churches to include an activity distinct from its other program offerings. It has taken the form of small group meetings in homes throughout the community in which members provide spiritual care one for another through Scripture and open communication. It is a splendid idea, provided that group members do communicate with one another rather than one person doing the talking and the rest listening. What is important is to develop an atmosphere of *mutual* spiritual care.

Caring for one another is an expression of love, something Jesus emphasized for all who would identify with him. Let's see how love ties in with mutual care.

What is it that Jesus said about love?

> A new command I give you: Love one another. As I have loved you, so you must love one another. By this all men will know that you are my disciples, if you love one another. (John 13:34–35)

He is saying that love shown in us toward others is the best possible verification of our discipleship, that we are followers of Christ. "By this all men will know that you are my disciples," he said. Or put another way, it is the best possible witness of our sincerity as Christians—a signal that points to our faith as one that works for the benefit of others. I think that is what Jesus had in mind. People will tend to give greater credence to biblical truths when they see them enacted in us through love. That is why we commonly step in to help victims of earthquakes, famines, and other natural disasters. We also show sensitivity toward people in their times of sorrow, sickness and death.

But how else do we follow Jesus' command to love? Does it have something to do with a more extensive sharing of our lives with one another? Could Jesus' statement about loving "As I have loved you" suggest what he had in mind? We will see. But let's not get ahead of ourselves.

Salvation: Prerequisite to Loving

The first step is to set love in motion by our own personal dependence on Christ for salvation. That is because we need a transformation which only Christ can give. Here is how the Bible declares it:

> Therefore, if anyone is in Christ, he is a new creation; the old has gone, the new has come! (2 Cor. 5:17)

Such is made possible when we accept Jesus' words about a spiritual birth (John 3:3–7), which then results in God's provision of the Holy Spirit to help us in a new adventure of living (Rom. 5:5). It is God's love implanted in us. It is not to be kept selfishly hidden there, but to be put to work for the benefit of others. Jesus explained it this way:

> No one lights a lamp and hides it in a jar or puts it under a bed. Instead, he puts it on a stand, so that those who come in can see the light. (Luke 8:16)

Having experienced this transformation by belief in Christ as Savior, we are in a position to start the process of truly loving others, just as Christ loved us. But we recognize that our situation isn't the same as that of the apostles. Jesus told them: "As I have loved you, so you must love one another." Although we have new birth in Christ, we have not been with Jesus in the flesh to experience the various ways he showed love toward those twelve with whom he walked and talked face to face.

Our recourse is to recognize the alternatives Jesus provided: (1) seeing him as recorded in the written record of the Bible; and, (2) experiencing his presence through the indwelling Holy Spirit who demonstrates in various ways God's love for us. If you are reading the Bible seriously, that is, contemplatively, so that you are letting God talk to you as discussed in the previous chapter, you will be experiencing his love expressed through Scripture. Likewise, if you take time to think about the different ways God has intervened in your life, you will understand the reality of his presence. But let's go on to Jesus' example of loving to see what it holds for us.

Jesus' Example

What does the Bible tell us about Jesus' show of love, in keeping with his statement, "As I have loved you?" We lack a record of all he said and did with his disciples. Such a document would consist of volumes, since it would cover events having taken place over the space of his three-year public ministry. But we do have some examples of Jesus' love as witnessed and recorded by his disciples—his compassion for the sick, his lament over the inhabitants of Jerusalem, his weeping over Lazarus' death, his identification with the sorrow and tears he saw among Lazarus' family and friends, and his pity for the sufferings of people in general. In this latter regard, see how Matthew expressed it:

> When he saw the crowds, he had compassion on them because they were harassed and helpless, like sheep without a shepherd. (Matt. 9:36)

Those examples refer to Jesus' love toward people in general. To be sure, his disciples witnessed it, and they were undoubtedly impacted by his tenderness as an example for them to follow. But how did he show his love specifically toward the chosen Twelve?

We see through the gospel accounts that Jesus' preoccupation with his disciples, aside from bringing them to a recognition of him as the Christ, was to teach them God's ways. He did it not only through words but by deeds. An outstanding case was his example of being a servant. He willingly washed his disciples feet to render an example of true servanthood. What show of love! God, the Creator of the universe, performing the lowly act of handling peoples' dusty and dirty feet. He did it to show them "the full extent of his love" (John 13:1).

Now we are getting down to measuring love—serving one another with such humility that it destroys any notions of superiority or pride. Jesus told his disciples:

> Do you understand what I have done for you? . . . Now that I, your Lord and Teacher, have washed your feet, you also should wash one another's feet. I have set for you an example that you should do as I have done for you. I tell you the truth, no servant is greater than his master, nor is a messenger greater than the one who sent him. Now that you know these things, you will be blessed if you do them. (John 13:12, 14–17)

That statement was hardly given to be taken in the literal sense of a foot-bathing ritual, but rather to emphasize something far more important—that love is shown through serving. And of course that serving is to be done no matter how ugly or repugnant the task.

But the greatest show of love is when one is willing to die for another. I suspect that in a marriage where true love exists, a spouse would readily give his or her life so that the other might live. If that were not so, I would question the strength of that love relationship. Christ exemplified the ultimate in love through his willingness to die for humanity. Do you remember his words?

> Greater love has no one than this, that he lay down his life for his friends. (John 15:13)

We see other ways in which Jesus showed his love toward the disciples. He did big things, like protecting them during the storm at sea; he did little things, like showing tenderness in preparing breakfast for them after their long night's toil at fishing.

When they landed, they saw a fire of burning coals with fish cooking, and some bread. Jesus said to them, "Come and have breakfast" (John 21:9, 12). How about that? The Master cooking fish over a fire for his friends.

We can speculate on other ways Jesus loved his disciples that go unrecorded. It was his godly nature to love, so he must have been tender toward them in times of hurt, sorrow, worry, and despair—things that crop up in life all the time. He also must have been concerned over providing for their continuing need of food and shelter. He surely cared for them when they got sick. He encouraged and gave support. He was empathic. He was there for them. He encouraged them in their walk with God. He *was* God, so he was love. And taking on the form of man he was able to understand the human need for love. Thus his commandment for us to love one another. When we follow it, we help attune people to God's love. And that is a marvelous accomplishment, because it brings joy to the hearts of many. Follow the Master in loving people.

Love is Serving

To follow Jesus' command to love one another, then, may very well stem on imitating his dedication to the service of others. Jesus expressed it by his concern for peoples' souls as well as for their physical comfort, spiritual wellness, and joy in this life. That is why he said in referring to himself as the shepherd who is concerned over his sheep.

> I have come that they may have life, and have it to the full. (John 10:10)

"Have it to the full." I like that. Could it mean that people out there are realizing only half or partial life? Christians included?

I, you, and all believers are his sheep. Like those helpless creatures depicted in Psalm 23, we have need for survival, we fear danger, we want comforting, we crave rest and contentment, we seek refreshing, all of which falls under the rubric of care. Jesus the Shepherd cares. He rescues, protects, guides and shows tenderness. Like cuddling a little lamb in his arms.

The Twenty-third Psalm ("The Lord is my Shepherd . . .") depicts those very characteristics. It reflects a show of tender care and love. But since Jesus isn't here bodily to present himself visibly as a provider of these needs, he indwells us through the Spirit who challenges us to be his ministers by caring and providing for others. Or as Paul put it: to "serve one another in love" (Gal. 5:13). In short, God uses us as ministers of love, love in action, that is. That reiterates Jesus' teaching of love in terms of servanthood.

The apostle John records an evening meal among Jesus and his disciples (John 13) which is similar to the account of the Lord's Supper in the Synoptic Gospels (Matthew, Mark and Luke). John's account, however, adds to it by relating the scene of Jesus washing his disciples' feet. Its inclusion wields a powerful message of humility tied to serving one another. Let it imprint on our minds that through that act of humility Jesus showed love by assuming a servant role. Does that mean love demands servanthood? I think so. It suggests a desire to serve with an attitude of humility. We can't separate love from humility.

The opposite of humility, of course, is pride. That ugly trait has interfered with love relationships from time immemorial. Marriage relationships suffer because of it. So do parent-children ties. When people hang on to pride, they upset loving relationships.

What message would you consider important to leave with those closest to you before your death? You might want to express for one last time your love for them. Jesus did the same thing, but in a slightly different way. He wanted them to love *one another*. You see, his children are important to him, and he wants us to assume a role in caring for them. It was his last charge to his disciples at a critical time, before his arrest and crucifixion. He exemplified it through the humble act of foot washing.

When allowed to blossom in one's life, loving others, according to Jesus, is the most powerful means of showing discipleship (John 13:35). In other words, if you want to draw someone closer to God, show love!

Putting love into practice by serving amounts to nothing less than performing acts of humility. When Jesus washed his disciples feet, humility was sticking out all over. But it didn't end there. Looking beyond that foot washing and the meal among Jesus and his disciples, we see the Son of God giving the ultimate example of humility—humbling himself through his substitutionary death. Hear Paul's words about what Jesus did:

> Taking the very nature of a servant . . . he humbled himself and became obedient to death—even death on a cross. (Phil. 2:7–8)

He not only loved us enough to die for us, but he did it in the most humiliating fashion—crucifixion. Paul wanted the Galatians to remember the ignominy of such a death:

> Christ redeemed us from the curse of the law by becoming a curse for us, for it is written: 'Cursed is everyone who is hung on a tree.' (Gal. 3:13) (Deut. 21:22–23)

Now there is the ultimate example of serving others—death, for the benefit of others, and to be cursed of the Father in the process. Being hung on a cross apparently signified God's rejection, which was probably the reason for Jesus crying out: "My God, my God, why have you forsaken me?" (Matt. 27:46).

What does this business of washing people's feet and dying in the place of others mean for us? Paul has the answer: Get with it and start serving one another! In other words, start copying Jesus!

> Having the same love, being one in spirit and purpose. Do nothing out of selfish ambition or vain conceit, but in humility consider others better than yourselves. Each of you should look not only to your own interests, but also to the interests of others. Your attitude should be the same as that of Christ Jesus. (Phil. 2:2–5)

Wow! We are to adopt Jesus' attitude? We are to get rid of any elements of pride that would make us think we are superior to others? We are to be concerned about the interests of others in addition to or maybe even beyond our own?

Are we followers of Christ? Then let's start serving others. According to the passage above, that means giving ourselves to the welfare of others. This takes us back to the formation and function of small care groups whereby members can actually serve one another.

Looking for Biblical Examples

Does the Bible contain any examples for ways to meet for mutual encouragement and service? It doesn't set forth a specific plan or formula to follow, but it does instruct on what *not* to do—allowing disorder, as in the Corinthian church (1 Cor. 14).[3] At the same time it gives a general but all important principle to follow: "Spur one another on to love and good deeds;" and, "Encourage one another" (Heb. 10:24–25). It is an admonition repeated in one of Paul's letters: "Encourage one another and build each other up" (1 Thess. 5:11).

The process points to the rationale for believers meeting together. Did you get it? It has to do with edifying and encouraging *one another*. I put the emphasis on those last two words because we tend to read the passage only in terms of edification and encouragement. We like to cite Sunday morning church as fulfilling those qualities because "the pastor does that," we say. Yes, he does. But that is one person edifying and encouraging everyone else; one person doing the talking, which is fine, because we need the wisdom the pastor has accumulated over years of study and personal experience with the Lord. But our preoccupation here is *mutual* encouragement, in providing spiritual care as Scripture describes it—*for one another*. That points to the active involvement of other people.

The Hebrews 10 passage is often used as a stimulus to get people to attend church: "Let us not give up meeting together" (Heb. 10:25). Passed over is the part regarding the *purpose* for meeting together "to spur one another on to love and good deeds." The critical concept tells us not to just meet together in whatever fashion, but to do it with a specific purpose. That objective is to grow in love for each other. It is growth in love toward God, to be sure, an objective we must never forget. But to stay true to the context, we see another important aspect of growth in love, one that is directed toward fellow believers.

Just as we tend to miss a critical goal of meeting together—growing in love toward brothers and sisters in Christ—so do we with the process. The latter requires *mutual* action. That means everyone doing their part—spurring *one another* to love and good deeds, as the Hebrews passage exhorts.

What is the big deal about multiple input? It has its rationale in the premise that all members, because of personal experiences and special abilities, contribute to meeting each other's needs. And it is not just a question of allowing a nice process to operate among whomever may wish to participate. Giving and receiving, that is, everyone encouraging each other, is what Scripture without doubt is addressing. It has in mind the well being of the entire church body.

The Church: The Body

Let's look at scriptural teaching about the body, because that is what the church is—a body of people, a living organism, not a building as tradition tends to define it. Paul compares the spiritual body, members of the church, with parts of the physical body:

> The body is a unit, though it is made up of many parts; and though all its parts are many, they form one body.

> So it is with Christ. For we were all baptized by one Spirit into one body—whether Jews or Greeks, slave or free—and we were all given one Spirit to drink. Now the body is not made up of one part but of many. If the foot should say, 'Because I am not a hand, I do not belong to the body,' it would not for that reason cease to be a part of the body. And if the ear should say, 'Because I am not an eye, I do not belong to the body,' it would not for that reason cease to be part of the body. If the whole body were an eye, where would the sense of hearing be? If the whole body were an ear, where would the sense of smell be? But in fact God has arranged the parts in the body, every one of them, just as he wanted them to be. If they were all one part, where would the body be? As it is, there are many parts, but one body. The eye cannot say to the hand, 'I don't need you!' And the head cannot say to the feet, 'I don't need you!' On the contrary, those parts of the body that seem to be weaker are indispensable, and the parts that we think are less honorable we treat with special honor. And the parts that are unpresentable are treated with special modesty, while our presentable parts need no special treatment. But God has combined the members of the body and has given greater honor to the parts that lacked it, so that there should be no division in the body, but that its parts should have equal concern for each other. If one part suffers, every part suffers with it; if one part is honored, every part rejoices with it. Now you are the body of Christ, and each one of you is a part of it. (1 Cor. 12:12–27)

Do you understand the message that the entire membership of the spiritual body, the church, is not only helpful in its overall function, but is actually necessary? That is what Paul declared, in the wisdom God gave him. Parts of the physical body must cooperate with other parts in order that all function properly. So it is with the spiritual body, the church. We can't do without the input of others if we are to enjoy the best in spiritual health.

We see a similar expression in Paul's Epistle to the Romans.

> Just as each of us has one body with many members, and these members do not all have the same function, so in Christ we who are many form one body, and each member belongs to all the others. We have different gifts, according to the grace given us. (Rom. 12:4–6)

Here Paul takes us one step further to show us God's provision for mutual service—different gifts. However, those God-given abilities must not be interpreted solely in terms of the highly esteemed ones of prophecy, teaching, or leadership. Paul cites those three gifts in the same Romans passage, but in the same breath he includes others also: serving (I am sure that doesn't just mean waiting on tables at church suppers); encouraging; generosity in contributing to the needs of others; and, showing mercy.

There is no question that some people do a better job of serving in these ways than do others. But everyone has the capacity to put them to work to some degree. God allows us to help each other by pulling experiences from our past. I may have just the right words to encourage someone who needs spiritual uplifting, for example, because I myself have undergone a similar experience, or because I was recently impressed in my Bible reading by a passage on that very need.

In yet another passage, Paul admonishes the Ephesians to acknowledge and take responsibility toward the spiritual body of which they are a part:

> From him (Christ) the whole body, joined and held together by every supporting ligament, grows and builds

> itself up in love, *as each part does its work.*" (emphasis mine) (Eph. 4:16)

Let's review the key elements of the above passages: (1) "its parts [the body] should have equal concern for one another;" (2) "each member belongs to all the others;" and, (3) "the whole body builds itself up in love, as each part does its work." In other words, believers have a responsibility for the welfare of each—to serve one another, which leads to growth in love one toward another. One person can't do it all, and we shouldn't expect him or her to. It demands multiple input with responsibility shared by all. We are indispensable, God says, to the spiritual growth and joy of *each other*.

To be sure, this exercise of love for the common welfare is at times expressed outside the church meeting, such as in comforting the sick and the bereaved, or meeting material needs. And how important all that is when suffering believers (and non-believers too), who find themselves in situations beyond their control, cry out for help. But there is more to communal care than that seen through these expressions of kindness. There is that other dimension in which Christians see the need for caring for one another in a host of spiritual needs, and to take steps to allow that process to take place, "as each part does its work."

From scriptural accounts we see that growth in love toward fellow believers was a vitality enjoyed by first century Christians. For example, the apostle Paul lauded the Colossian and Thessalonian churches saying,

> We always thank God . . . because we have heard of your faith in Christ Jesus and of *the love you have for all the saints.* (emphasis mine) (Col. 1:3–4)

> We ought always to thank God for you, brothers, and rightly so, because your faith is growing more and more, and *the love every one of you has for each other is increasing*. (emphasis mine) (2 Thess. 1:3)

Paul wished that our love for one another be intense:

> May the Lord make your love *overflow* for each other. (emphasis mine) (1 Thess. 3:12)

Peter saw it as "loving one another *deeply*" (emphasis mine) (1 Peter 1:22).

Can you imagine what those descriptions mean and what they require? Look at them again. Can provision for this kind of relationship be put into effect among Christians today? Meeting together in small groups is proving to be an effective means of doing that. We find its roots in the house meetings of early Christians. That is alluded to in various scriptural passages (Acts 2:46) (Acts 20:20) (Rom. 16) (1 Cor. 16:19) (Col. 4:15) (Philem. 2). Such an environment has its advantages for encouraging close relationships, because small numbers of people are conducive to intimate sharing. I should point out, however, that early Christians also came together in places allowing for larger meetings (Acts 2:46). I want to make that clear, should you be tempted to go off the deep end to exclude large group gatherings. Those first century believers saw the spiritual benefits of meeting in small intimate groups, so they provided for it. That is the point—not emphasizing the setting itself, but rather the purpose for meeting together, which will suggest the setting.

Creating Care Groups

As of now I will refer to small groups as "care groups," for want of a better name. Some churches follow the path of care groups by creating house meetings throughout their communities. I suppose you could do it differently by making available the church plant for such gatherings, although it lacks the warmth and intimacy of a living room. Whatever the physical setting, the point is to provide for open sharing cultivated for growth in love for one another. That may not be done if an impersonal process is followed. The latter is a throw back to mere acquisition of knowledge, so often seen in Bible classes. Care must be taken not to let mere knowledge of Bible content become the focal point.

The start up of a care group movement might seem to some as just another church activity. Church members probably won't get excited about it unless they have previous knowledge of the impact it carries on participants. That is a challenge for the church leadership to make known.

How might a small care group meeting function? We don't want to create a spectator scene in which group members just listen while the leader does all the talking. The wise leader (sharing facilitator) sets the tone for multiple input as he or she maintains the premise that all need each other, that all have something to say that others need, and consequently that all be encouraged to share. It is a process of mutual responsibility leading to fulfillment of Christ's command to love one another. And that love is not just an idea to be mouthed. It is action.

The Sharing Content

What then is to be the content? More spiritually mature groups may leave it to its individual members to define the content, as they come prepared to share the various ways God is working in their lives. For example, you may:

(1) read a verse or group of verses from the Bible, and tell why that Scripture has been especially meaningful to you for the week;
(2) share a personal experience in which God's presence was evident. What he has done for you may be just what he wants to do for others through your shared experience;
(3) sing a hymn or chorus, and relate why its message is important to you;[4]
(4) voice a personal need (frustration, discouragement, disappointment, etc.), to which others may respond through spiritual insight and/or prayer;
(5) voice a personal praise or thanksgiving;
(6) announce a prayer request, which the group will address together (as well as each member making intercessory prayer at home throughout the week); [5] and,
(7) allow activities to flow naturally, which in essence means yielding to the leading and direction of the Holy Spirit as to what and when certain things are to take place. That may mean putting aside previously planned procedures you intended to follow.

Should you wish to use a more structured approach, you may want to select certain materials as a base for discussion. For example, a predetermined Bible passage, a book on spiritual living, or a workbook may serve the purpose. (Check your local Christian bookstore for discussion-enabling materials.) This approach places greater responsibility on the group leader to search for ways to incite members to enter into the discussion, not necessarily pushing personalizing at first, but always probing for that to happen. Success will rest largely on the leader's skill toward that end, and of course on his or her setting the tone by personal example. As more people share personal experiences, the group will recognize the blessings of that sharing, and will feel responsibility for personal input for the benefit of all.

Another approach is simply to discuss books of the Bible (e.g., one of the Gospels, or an Epistle). Care must be given, however, to emphasize application rather than acquisition of knowledge. Otherwise, you end up with just another Bible class.

I am talking about a very special type of meeting where all that is said and done reflects God's working as personally experienced by the participants. You might react by saying, "If that's the criterion for participation, no one will say anything." Not so! I am talking about grace, faith, and love in action, which expresses spiritual concerns and biblical truths that everyone has experienced to some degree. It is a question of directing participants' awareness to the ongoing experiences God brings into their lives. The voicing of these personal events demonstrates the Word of God in action—encouraging listeners to apply Scripture experientially rather than as an accumulation of facts. And the more we participate in this personalizing, the more we attune ourselves to God's interaction with us in our daily activities, which forms a basis for contributing to the sharing process.

By the way, a part of our makeup as social beings is the desire to use our strengths in some way or another to render service to others. Reading the Bible is of course important for our own spiritual nurturing, but eventually it must have an outlet. Otherwise, it runs the danger of losing its appeal. Delving into Scripture by reading, studying, meditating, and even memorizing takes a good degree of personal discipline. If there is no outlet for sharing our learning, discouragement can set in. Compare it to the physical of eating without exercise. You may say, "Oh, but you have an outlet in witnessing to the lost." That is certainly an important outcome, but it fulfills only one part of our obligation to minister. The other part is our ministry to fellow saints.

The whole spiritual process of extracting strength from the Bible is similar to the physical: continuous energy intake without output makes for an unhealthy and frustrated individual. We seem to have a natural inclination and even need to share our learning experiences with others. That compulsion seems to be part of our human nature, maybe because of the joy it gives us to help others.

I remind you that I am not just talking about intake of knowledge. That of course is a part of the learning process. But what is important is how knowledge becomes a reality through application. I think we all distinguish between sharing truths that are simply knowledge-based versus those reflecting personal application. The former, be it presented in the form of a sermon, a devotional, or just a minute or two of talking, lacks the dynamic thrust to affect the listeners if the speaker gives no evidence of having applied it experientially. It takes on characteristics of mere human analysis. But application, when related to the sharer's personal experience, has a power that challenges the listeners' receptivity to the reality of God's intimacy.

In other words, it is not a question of merely *talking* about concepts of comfort, peace, joy, and other forms of blessings. We *show* them as fruits that blossom in the reality of our very own lives. Herein is the encouragement and edification I believe Scripture tells Christians to practice with one another. It is spiritual sharing that packs a wallop.

It is my experience that in a meeting where this kind of sharing takes place, a time of interconnected activities will tend to flow. People participate as they see it appropriate from what went on before. Their participation will be stimulated by any of the activities I have listed as possibilities for care group content, and there will tend to be a natural flowing unity of discourse and activity that increases meaning for the listeners. The message that members share will often instigate someone picking up on it with his or her own insights. I mention this as an added blessing that comes naturally and that gives a greater sense of relevance to all that is said and done. It isn't something, however, that we should strive to bring about artificially.

To participate actively in this kind of care is a strong stimulus for each person to be walking with God in its various facets throughout the week (such as Bible reading/study, prayer, meditation, sharing the gospel with others, and observing and thanking God for his involvement in our daily experiences). It gives us content to talk about. It likewise forces us to evaluate our own daily walk in terms of whether it is of any worth sharing. If we are hard pressed to come up with anything to talk about, what does that tell us of our daily ongoing communion with the Lord?

I have taken the risk of giving examples of how a care group might function. You should understand that I have done so in the spirit of providing only guidelines. It isn't the only way for care groups to meet. Each group will have to experiment on its own to learn the best way to function to meet the needs of its members. At first, the meeting may appear clumsy. People will not be sure how to participate. But as the major purpose of the meeting is kept in mind, and all are responsible members, the group will learn to function smoothly and in tune with the Spirit's leading. What is important to remember is that the care group's purpose is for all to encourage and edify *one another*. If that concept is lost, the group loses its uniqueness and dynamism; it becomes merely another gathering of Christians with only one or maybe a couple of people doing the talking. And people start accepting that kind of procedure because they believe they best be quiet in deference to those more verbal.

Much of this has to do with our preparedness to allow God to use us in his ministry among the body of believers. It is an exciting venture. That is the message portrayed to first-century believers.

> Do not get drunk on wine, which leads to debauchery. Instead, be filled with the Spirit. Speak to one another with psalms, hymns and spiritual songs. Sing and make music in your hear to the Lord, always giving thanks to God the Father for everything. (Eph. 5:18–20)

The passage has two important components: our cooperation with the Holy Spirit to direct our lives; and, our using that "filling" in helping each other spiritually. Let's see below how that works.

Filled with the Spirit

"Filled with the Spirit" in the above passage is represented by the Greek word *pleroo,* whose meaning has to do with submission to the Spirit. This is a different scenario from other New Testament references about the Spirit's filling which resulted in miraculous abilities, as in tongues and prophecy. Could "submission" in the Ephesians passage be tied to a deliberate effort on our part to help one another through more ordinary means rather through supernatural events such as were seen in the first-century church?

How do we follow the command to be filled with the Spirit? Some people are so obsessed with being given the "filling" that they pray and wait for its occurrence. We get a totally different point of view by comparing the Ephesians passage with that of Colossians. Both are similar except for one crucial point: *be filled with the Spirit* (Eph. 5:18) and *Let the word of Christ dwell in you richly* (Col. 3:16). Here is the exact wording of the two passages side by side.

Ephesians 5:18–20	Colossians 3:16–17
Do not get drunk on wine, which leads to debauchery. Instead, *be filled with the Spirit.* Speak to one another with psalms, hymns and spiritual songs. Sing and make music in your heart to the Lord, always giving thanks to God the Father for everything (emphasis mine).	*Let the word of Christ dwell in you richly* as you teach and admonish one another with all wisdom, and as you sing psalms, hymns and spiritual songs with gratitude in your hearts to God . . . giving thanks to God the Father (emphasis mine).

Is *being filled with the Spirit* (Ephesians) synonymous with *letting the word of Christ dwell in you richly*? (Colossians). Their similar outcomes of rendering spiritual help (*speaking to one another, and teaching and admonishing one another*) point to their likeness. How then do we allow that to happen?

Since the Spirit has an intimate relationship with us by living within us, he surely desires that we attune ourselves to his communication. That seems to be what Paul was driving at when saying we shouldn't be under the control of wine but instead be filled with (submitted to, under the control of) the Spirit. Putting the two passages together, we see the relationship between the Spirit and the Bible. In one instance it talks in terms of the Spirit as the dominating force, while in another, the word of Christ. Since we have the Scripture in its completeness, and it is Spirit (John 6:63), we can extend God's communication to people by utilizing it. Indeed the Bible is a set of holy writings inspired by the Spirit for our growth in love (2 Tim. 3:16–17). As we use the Spirit's words we unleash their power on the lives of our listeners.

That is precisely what happens when we come together to meet each other's needs. Take special notice of the above references as they both talk about helping *one another*. It is *mutual* spiritual care. If we let that slip by unnoticed, we miss the whole point of this discussion.

We must keep in mind that these are characteristics all believers are to exhibit toward their brothers and sisters in Christ. It is helping one another meet the spiritual needs confronting us daily. It is a beautiful privilege, but also an awesome responsibility.

Love: The Bible's Main Emphasis

Let's be reminded that Jesus' main charge to Christians is to love one another. It constitutes a command above all other commands. Indeed, it is one that fulfills all other commands Jesus gave:

> A new command I give you: Love one another. As I have loved you, so you must love one another. By this all men will know that you are my disciples if you love one another. (John 13:34)

Paul said:

> Serve one another in love. (Gal. 5:13)

Paul also said:

> May the Lord make your love increase and overflow for each other. (1 Thess. 3:12)

Peter said:

> Now that you have purified yourselves by obeying the truth so that you have sincere love for the brethren, love one another deeply, from the heart. (1 Peter 1:22)

John said:

> Dear friends, let us love one another, for love comes from God. Everyone who loves has been born of God, and knows God. (1 John 4:7)

These represent but a few examples that emphasize the love we are to have for each other. Their message is crucial: love toward one another follows the examples given by Jesus and the apostles: love is serving; love is of such magnitude that, when shown, it overflows among others; love is deep, not superficial; and, love is a testimony of being born of God.

We keep saying we want to be like Jesus. Well, there it is—loving one another. The Bible is replete with instruction on loving. It is its main message for believers.

How to Love

Now we must come to grips with how we do it? Certainly we don't love simply by acknowledging it intellectually for the sake of knowledge. We must put it into practice. And that means we must learn how to love. The process begins by committing ourselves to those whom we are to love. That is done by spending time with them, just as we learn to love God by spending time with him.

In Chapter Four on *Loving God*, I suggested this concept along with the notion of listening to God. We must do the same with one another—learn to listen. That is the way we get to really know our fellow brothers and sisters, and it is of course quite impossible to listen without allowing them to speak.

So it makes sense to establish an environment in which saints gather in an intimate, sharing atmosphere, one in which they glean spiritual insight from the lives of one another. That environment will allow us to reveal our joys, hurts, hopes, aspirations, victories, defeats, doubts and confusions, and all that is taking place in our lives for which tender care can be given. It comes about as we identify with what a brother or sister is experiencing as we see the same or similar happening in our lives. Empathy results, and it makes for our love toward that person to grow. It is a love that binds.

But that makes us vulnerable. Are we prepared to take off our masks and be genuine? It can be done when we agree to commit ourselves to one another in an atmosphere of trust, all toward the end goal of growing in genuine love for one another. But we must understand that trust doesn't happen automatically. It requires a visible show of concern, as in caring for a sick brother or sister, or in being a friend to one who has been unjustly vilified, or in spending time with one whose spouse has just died. Trust is earned over time. It can precede fellowship in a care group, or it can be the result of it.

I am talking about developing deep relationships, even as Peter encouraged us to "love one another deeply." We tend to fear such ties because we know that personal responsibilities are involved. We have trouble with selfishness, especially in terms of time, and so we find it hard to give ourselves to others. Then we are troubled about openness, because we will have to stop projecting images of self-sufficiency and start revealing our true selves. We can go along with sharing our joys, but we shudder at the thought of revealing loneliness, failures, fears, and hurts. We readily share with others by attending to their physical needs of food, clothing, and the like. Just pull out the checkbook and make a contribution. No real personal involvement. Love oversimplified.

We can't be impersonal with love. Love deals with emotional needs. Why should we deal with them? "Everyone has them," you may be thinking. "Leave the emotions alone and eventually they will fade and extinguish themselves," you may argue. Some of them will, probably most. But why give them opportunity to take away our joy, albeit temporarily? Even the most minor troubles keep us from enjoying God's provisions of peace, rest, and security. That is where Christians come to the rescue of one another, sharing our personal experience of God's presence for mutual encouragement.

Unless we incorporate this idea of spending time with one another as a prerequisite to growth in love, our relationships will likely remain minimal and superficial. Look at relations between husbands and wives. Spouses grow in love toward each other as they live together (provided of course they are open with each other). They learn of each other's needs. They communicate. They sacrifice for each other. Love to them is a commitment.

In a similar vein it is with the Christian who wants to find a mutually supporting relationship with fellow believers. We have lost this concept within the Church. If we are to take seriously Christ's command to love, we must provide the means to see it accomplished. You may say, "I don't need to do that in a group. I can do it with my spouse, or with my fiancée." That may be beneficial, but not in the same sense as getting God's input from the rest of the body. Let's not forget the critical nature of each member of the body being needed for the proper functioning of the body. That is a scriptural declaration.

In keeping with my reference to love as the main emphasis of the New Testament, I remind you of Paul's love chapter to the Corinthians:

> If I speak in the tongues of men and of angels, but have not love, I am only a resounding gong or a clanging cymbal. If I have the gift of prophecy and can fathom all mysteries and all knowledge, and if I have a faith that can move mountains, but have not love, I am nothing. If I give all I possess to the poor and surrender my body to the flames, but have not love, I gain nothing. Love is patient, love is kind. It does not envy, it does not boast, it is not proud. It is not rude, it is not self-seeking, it is not easily angered, it keeps no record of wrongs. Love does not delight in evil but rejoices with the truth. It always protects, always trusts, always hopes, always perseveres. Love never fails. (1 Cor. 13:1–8)

These verses record characteristics of love, first in the positive and then in the negative. In the positive, love exhibits patience and kindness, it is protecting, trusting, and persevering. In the negative: love doesn't allow envy, boasting, pride, rudeness, selfishness, anger, or vindictiveness. Try that hat on for size! How many of us measure up consistently?

Someone made a good suggestion for personalizing the Corinthians passage above—substitute the word *love* with *I:* as in *I am patient, I am kind, I do not envy, I do not boast, I am not proud, I am not rude, I am not self-seeking, I am not easily angered, I do not keep a record of wrongs,* etc. How's that for a lesson in humility.

Embedded in the above list are concerns of all of us. I think that may be why both Jesus and Paul defined loving one's neighbor as loving one's self. It suggests treating people in the same way we would like them to treat us. Let's reflect for a moment on what that might entail. We want to be accepted, appreciated, and recognized; likewise we crave affection and empathy; and, we hope people will be forgiving, tender, and sensitive to our feelings. You can add to the list. The point is that these items help define love. The simple application of love is found in the following: Do I want people to treat me with patience, understanding, acceptance, appreciation, etc.? Then I had better start treating them that way too. It is living out the golden rule of doing to others what you would have them do to you.

Our challenge is to apply the wonderful love chapter from Corinthians to loving brothers and sisters in Christ. It is putting love into action. But if we are to do it, it seems fair to say that it must concern issues we all face in the process of daily living. That represents love in reality, not in theory. What is happening in our lives is important for all to hear in preparation for dealing with similar events that may come about in their lives. That is one of the ways God has given us to help one another. It is one of his provisions to sustain us, indeed to bless us. And more, by our love we will be showing ourselves as his disciples (John 13:35). Do you remember? According to Jesus, there is no greater testimony to the world about the truth of Christianity and our commitment to it than our show of love one toward another. Giving love is the grand witness of our faith.

Building Unity

There is another reference to loving fellow believers that I believe appropriate to this discussion—Jesus' prayer for our Christian unity: "So that they may be one as we are one," he cried out to the Father (John 17:11). Just as we tend to lack the slightest concern about growing in love toward one another, so we are guilty of gross disunity across the gamut of Christendom. I am not advocating a surrender to basic doctrine on salvation through Christ in order to create a false sense of oneness. But we seem to be at each others throats on so many other matters that will be of doubtful importance when we get to heaven. Standing there together with fellow saints, no one will be so brazen as to say: "What are you doing here? You weren't baptized by immersion." Or, "Hey, how did you make it here? You don't speak in tongues." Or, "Well whaddaya know. You divorced your spouse and remarried, and yet you're here." Or, "I don't understand how you got in. You're of such-and-such a church or denomination." And on and on it could go.

The point is that those ideas we dogmatically give such credence to on earth will disappear in the blink of an eye when we stand before the throne of the Almighty. And if you are thinking, "No! Those people won't be in heaven," then you are in the worst of shape. And we wonder why the world scoffs at Christianity. Let Jesus' words ring in our ears as he interceded for others (us) in addition to his chosen twelve.

> I pray also for those who will believe in me through their message, that all of them may be one, Father, just as you are in me and I am in you. May they also be in us *so that the world may believe that you have sent me.* (emphasis mine) (John 17:20–21)

"So that the world may believe that you have sent me." Does that sound familiar? Compare it with Jesus' earlier teaching when he said we should love one another *so that the world will know we are his disciples.* In one instance he spoke of love; in another he emphasized unity. He connected both with the witness they carry to onlookers.

The critical question in all of this is: How do you suppose we are going to be a witness to the world of the truth of Christianity unless we are united? And how do you suppose we are to experience unity unless we get serious about loving one another?

The Indwelling Spirit: A Stimulus to Love

Although I have given you a challenge to take steps to grow in love toward fellow believers, I will not make the mistake of having you believe it is accomplished through self-effort. Good news! We have help to set things in motion. It is done through a very special unction of the Holy Spirit, who comes to live in us to make us a holy temple in God's sight. Paul explains,

> For we are the temple of the living God. As God has said: I will live with them and walk among them, and I will be their God, and they will be my people. (2 Cor. 6:16)

The Holy Spirit is a unifying force in making all Christians one very special people in God's eyes.

> Because you are sons, God has sent the Spirit of his Son into our hearts, the Spirit who calls out, 'Abba, Father.' (Gal. 4:6)

That speaks to me in the sense that if God indwells believers and considers them special (as sons and daughters), then I have the obligation to view them as special too. After all, why would I want to have an attitude toward them which differs from that of my Lord?

The Holy Spirit represents an identifying feature of our possession by God. That fact has serious implications about my attitude toward and treatment of other believers. If I show anger or bitterness, I hear God crying out, "What are you doing to my child? I have made you all a part of my family. You are an important part of my household. Don't you understand the implications of that?"

A second thought in this regards is the special role of the Holy Spirit in identifying believers for the coming day of their redemption, their transfer from earth to heaven. It is an identification made through faith at the very moment we first believed the gospel message. Here are the exact words:

> And you also were included in Christ when you heard the word of truth, the gospel of your salvation. Having believed, you were marked in him with a seal, the promised Holy Spirit, who is a deposit guaranteeing our inheritance until the redemption of those who are God's possession—to the praise of his glory. (Eph. 1:13–14)

This passage reminds us again of the special status of Christians in God's eyes, a status that sets us apart from the rest of the world by a marking of the Spirit. We can't, of course, see that Spirit, but we know he is there, because we observe him (dare I say "feel" him?) working in our lives. Paul testified to the fact that the Spirit in many different ways tells us we belong to God. (Rom. 8:16–27) (1 Cor. 2:9–12). Do not restrict God by thinking that the Spirit is there only to remind us of our salvation, as important as that is. He is also there to administer God's blessings on us, to show us God's love and care in all of life's circumstances.

I don't minimize the Spirit's importance in reminding me of my secure position in Christ. The Scripture speaks of the Holy Spirit in that regard as "guaranteeing our inheritance," that is, God's acceptance of us for eternal life with him. All the more reason why we should treat each other as special. We will be living together in heaven someday. We will be standing together before our Lord who bought us with his life, and he will treat each of us as equally special. Will we be ashamed in heaven as we remember the way we treated the person who may end up next to us?

This has had special meaning to me as far back as my teenage years. Not long after I came to grips with believing the gospel message, I worked on the assembly line of the local General Electric plant. I was enthusiastic about my newfound faith and was eager to find other believers with whom I could identify. During the rest break I saw a young man down the line reading the Bible. I figured that anyone doing that under such circumstances had to be a Christian. So I walked over to introduce myself as a brother in Christ. To my astonishment, he hadn't the slightest interest in conversing or even knowing who I was. I said to myself, "If this guy's a believer, what a gross inconsistency to be reading the Bible and yet being rude to another Christian seeking friendship." I don't know what caused him to act that way, but from that day on I resolved never to view a believer in Christ as common or ordinary. The world often rejects us. But a fellow Christian?

If Christians are special to God, they should be special to us too. In my opinion, that demands a special love relationship with them. We should not take one another for granted. It is inconsistent with our family relationship in Christ. Indeed, it is an affront to God. We are his children, brothers and sisters in the faith, which is an extraordinary standing that should affect our behavior toward each other. After all, we will be living together for eternity in heaven where our Father will love each of us as very special people. Meanwhile, as I await that glorious event, Jesus' words are ringing in my ears:

> As I have loved you, so you must love one another. By this all men will know that you are my disciples, if you love one another. (John 13:34)

Loving fellow Christians. That is the theme of this chapter. Let's recall again John's account of a meal among Jesus and his disciples at which the Master, in washing his disciples' feet, made two life-guiding principles characteristic of love: 1) humility, and, 2) servanthood. Following the washing ritual, Jesus said to them:

> I have set you an example that you should do as I have done for you. I tell you the truth, no servant is greater than his master, nor is a messenger greater than the one who sent him. Now that you know these things, you will be blessed if you do them. (John 13:15–17)

Now let's understand what is embedded in that passage. The first and most obvious is that Jesus set an example for us on the characteristics of true love, and that by following him we will reap its blessings. What do you suppose those blessings are? Putting love into action results in joy, for both the receiver and the giver. Are you walking about glum? Does your face seem so long and mulish as if to say you could eat your oats out of a milk carton? Start loving others and get joy!

The second challenge displayed in John's gospel is that we get off our high horses and start practicing humility. Who do we think we are, holding on to superiority attitudes? Jesus' admonition is that *he* is *the* master, we are just servants. Let's not forget it!

Following John's account, we see events we connect with the Passover feast—Jesus' prediction of betrayal, the partaking of bread and wine, and Jesus' reference to his upcoming death. That is the scene the Apostle depicts when he quotes Jesus' famous words of his new command that we love one another.

I have repeated the account of the scene in order to impress its message upon your heart. In that evening meal, we see an interesting inclusion in John's account—Jesus taking advantage of his final hours with his disciples to remind them of the most important thing he wanted them to remember—to learn to love one another by taking on humility and a servant attitude. It amounts to putting love into action. It involves considering others better than ourselves (Phil. 2:3), and at the same time it counteracts a host of undesirable traits such as selfishness, pride, vanity, jealousy, anger, contempt, and other negatives that tend to crop up and interfere with our dealings with people—behaviors that hurt us as well as cause our Lord grief. Wow! Look what the practice of love accomplishes.

Love is the trait Jesus expressed above all others throughout his ministry as well as in his last instructions to the Twelve. Why did he zero in on love? *Because it is the central issue regarding a relationship with our heavenly Fa-*

ther and with human beings. We must make it a part of our lives as we interact with fellow saints. In the same breath, Jesus said he would help his disciples do just that—to put love into action (John 14). He would not leave us to struggle with it on our own; he would send the Holy Spirit to indwell us to be our helper. It underscores the uniqueness and special status of his children, of which we should take heed in our relationship with one another.

I have suggested an application of Jesus' command about loving one another through the formation of small care groups. It is obvious, however, that growth in love through such a setting is a somewhat limited scenario in the sense that it involves only members of a particular group. But it isn't quite as limiting as it may seem, since it has a multiplication process embedded in its make-up whereby many groups blossom from one single group. This is done as groups grow in number and then split to make way for new members, which is done to maintain smallness for facilitating intimate sharing, but also to create the formation of other groups which expands the ministry. Although we are not getting to love everyone deeply outside of our own particular care group, we are facilitating it among others as more groups organize and function.

Through a care group, we provide a means for developing the deep love one toward another that the apostle Peter addressed. It is the most demanding level of love, yet one that seems necessary for enhancing real strength, comfort, and joy in our Christian lives.

This kind of communal activity takes on another dimension from love engendered in the traditional Sunday morning church service. I hope you will not hold to that latter activity—worship—as important as it is, as fulfilling your Christian responsibilities. To be sure, worship is a way of showing our love toward God. But it is only one way.

There are many others ways, and they are so crucial to the well-being of the church body. They demand active involvement that calls for servanthood—giving ourselves to others—which Jesus defined in his command to love one another.

The second application I have suggested is that of going beyond the small group and loving all Christians. It is obviously love on a less intimate level than the first, considering the lesser contact time involved and the tendency for lesser intimacy. But it is a love that Jesus addressed in the sense of our commonality as brothers and sisters in the faith, one in which acts of compassion and generosity are in order. Furthermore, God sees us as special people by indwelling us with his presence—the Father, Son and Holy Spirit making their home in us. That presence is a divine mark that says we are favored as God's children through Jesus Christ. We must love one another for that very reason—to reflect the same special attitude that God has toward all who believe in his Son. Honoring Christians is in effect honoring the God who lives within them. What a splendid idea to keep in mind when negative thoughts toward a fellow believer start entering our minds.

The third application of love comes in the next chapter. It involves what I believe to be Jesus' command to love in an even wider sense, to include all people in general, no matter what their faith. We of course exercise such love through sharing materially. But that is not all. There is a spiritual element to it also. It might be characterized as Christian tenderness or compassion. Let's see what it entails.

CHAPTER 6

Loving All People

"Love your neighbor as yourself."

Galatians 5:14

Compassion

In this chapter I refer to people no matter what their religious faith or lack of it. The driving force for loving them I see as compassion, which includes a feeling for their physical and material welfare as well as for their spiritual well being. God proclaimed it through the prophet Zechariah:

> This is what the Lord Almighty says: '. . . show mercy and compassion to one another.' (Zech. 7:9)

Through television and other media we are informed of a multitude of needs throughout the world—monumental suffering caused by war, disease, famine, earthquakes, and other disasters. Christians have a role to play here. If we need an urging from Scripture, we are told to do good to everyone (Gal. 5:10) and also to share with those in need (Rom. 12:13).

The wisdom from Proverbs tells us of God's pleasure over our compassion toward people, with specific emphasis on the poor, who are always among us.

> He who is kind to the poor lends to the Lord. (Prov. 19:17)

The second part of the verse speaks of it as a loan with the promise of repayment:

> And he will reward him for what he has done.

That is not necessarily to be interpreted as monetary reward, nor should that even be our incentive. But the message seems to be that God will bless us in one way or another for our compassion. That demonstrates the importance God gives toward helping the poor. James gets specific in identifying recipients of our care as he reminds us,

> Look after orphans and widows in their distress. (James 1:27)

Orphans can not take care of their own needs. They are helpless. Someone must come to their rescue. The same applies to widows, who are often left without financial means to care for themselves. We don't have to look far to find people in desperate need of help. If we are in love with God, we will want to reflect that love toward others, to show his compassion, just as Jesus did in the many instances of feeding the multitudes and of healing the sick and disabled. I remind you of the parable Jesus gave about the

Good Samaritan. It has to do with showing compassion, all in the context of loving God and fellow human beings. It involves a man on the way to Jericho who fell prey to robbers, was beaten, and left in miserable condition. A Jewish priest passing by avoided him, and so did a Levite.

> But a Samaritan, as he traveled, came where the man was; and when he saw him, he took pity on him. He went to him and bandaged his wounds, pouring on oil and wine. Then he put the man on his own donkey, took him to an inn and took care of him. The next day he took out two silver coins and gave them to the innkeeper. 'Look after him,' he said, 'and when I return, I will reimburse you for any extra expense you may have.' (Luke 10:33–35)

Jesus told this story in answer to "an expert in the law" who, scheming to test him, asked what he had to do to inherit eternal life. Jesus replied with an appropriate question to this "expert."

> What is written in the Law? . . . How do you read it? (v. 26)

The man answered,

> 'Love the Lord your God with all your heart and with all your soul and with all your strength and with all your mind and, Love your neighbor as yourself.' (v. 27)

Jesus responded,

> 'You have answered correctly . . . Do this and you will live.' (v. 28)

But the clincher was the man's follow-up question, when he asked: Who is my neighbor? (v. 29) He seemed determined to try to best Jesus in the dialogue. It precipitated the story of the Good Samaritan.

What is it all about? Jesus wasn't teaching that one gets to heaven by doing good deeds. Rather, he got the guy thinking in the context of his specialty—the law—the substance of which is to love God with sincerity and to prove it by being compassionate. If we look carefully at the sum of Jesus' teachings, we will see it continually saying love, love, love. Love is sticking out all over. The law expert knew that the crux of the law was love. But he wasn't practicing it, as can be seen by his smart-alecky question: "And who is my neighbor?" (v. 29) We, on the other hand, know better. Right? Hmmm. Showing our love for God by loving our fellow man is a lesson we all need reminding of. It is love in action, not just words. That is what Jesus meant when, after teaching his disciples about love, he said,

> Now that you know these things, you will be blessed if you do them. (John 13:17)

John's epistle says essentially the same thing—practicing love, not just talking about it (1 John 3:18).

As we put love into practice, we show God's compassion. That may take the form of donation of material goods, friendship, comfort, volunteerism or other benevolent acts. I am reminded of Isaiah's advice to the Israelites in this regard. They fasted and humbled themselves before God, but it didn't result in God's presence they so desperately sought. Why didn't God come to them? Because their actions were hypocritical. They put on airs of being religious by fasting, while at the same time failing to attend to those in need. What a lesson for us in our religious activity!

What precisely was God expecting of them?

> Is it not to share your food with the hungry and to provide the poor wanderer with shelter—when you see the naked, to clothe him? (Isa. 58:7)

I like God's tenderness when he told them that their concern for the needs of others would result in his show of concern toward them in *their* time of need:

> Then you will call, and the Lord will answer; you will cry for help, and he will say: *Here am I.* (emphasis mine) (Isa. 58:9)

There is another point to consider. We can be sure that God uses every charitable deed of ours to bring people closer to him. The ultimate result he desires, of course, is that people acknowledge him for salvation. God is so tender toward people that he wants them to be saved and to come to a knowledge of the truth, wrote Paul (1 Tim. 2:3). He wants his creation to enjoy the glory of an eternity in heaven as well as the earthly blessings that come from a son/daughter relationship with him. Those blessings come out of his grace and love, coupled with our faith. They involve such things as joyous surprises in life, and even intimate whispers of comfort and peace in times of sorrow or distress. We play a role in this regard by heeding Jesus' commission to take the gospel to the world. In a sense it seems strange that he has given us this responsibility, for in his omnipotence he doesn't need us to spread his message of love and grace. Yet he has chosen to take that route, to make us responsible to do it. That is his choice. Anyway, being recipients of his marvelous grace through salvation, why would we not want to share it with others? It is the ultimate demonstration of compassion.

We see the examples of the apostles and of other first-century Christians spreading the Good News of Christ, and we are challenged to follow their example. But aside from becoming missionaries overseas, how do we go about it right where we are?

Witnesses of Salvation

The typical answer that has been drummed into our heads is simply to get out and witness. We interpret that in different ways: Should we share the gospel boldly with everyone within our daily activities, or should we reserve it for those who in some way indicate spiritual interest? Should we create opportunities, or should we wait for God to open doors? Should we be compulsive during a conversation, or should we first establish friendship and wait for an opening, an appropriate time to talk seriously? And above all, is the task our doing or God's? Answers to these questions have ramifications as to how our witness is received, perhaps with anger and rejection, or with reflection and deliberation, or with outright joy and acceptance.

Sharing the gospel with others, or witnessing, as some call it, not only brings people to Christ for salvation, but also changes their lives and those of their families too. How often have we heard of people ruined by such habits as alcohol abuse, drugs, gambling, and sexual immorality who were able to turn themselves around through faith in Christ. God gives power to set lives straight.

My own experience on the effects of people speaking the Gospel goes back to my youth in Erie, Pennsylvania, where my mother operated a beauty salon. One day two customers spoke to her about Jesus. Curious, she took up their invitation to visit their church. She discovered for the first time God's love for her through Christ. That resulted eventually in my salvation too, as well as that of the rest of the family. All because of two women who wanted to share Jesus.

Two faithful witnesses. I have often wondered what kind of persons I and my siblings would be today had it not been for the love of those ladies who shared Christ with my mother.

I have been profoundly affected by that story—through my own salvation, of course, but also by the lesson it teaches to be a faithful witness for my Lord wherever I go. There are people out there whom God wishes to reach with his message of grace and love. And he wants me to be his courier. Just as those two women who helped my mother understand and receive God's gift through Jesus.

I also want to include here *my* experience in sharing the faith with others. Unfortunately, it is not a positive one as that mentioned above. Shortly after becoming a Christian, I got caught up with a group of believers who viewed witnessing as a duty, a kind of law that must be followed to measure one's spirituality. I was asked to join the group in handing out gospel tracts. For my hesitancy I was rebuffed and made to feel guilty. "What's the matter with you? Are you ashamed of the gospel?" they unkindly suggested as they quoted Romans 1:16 ("I am not ashamed of the gospel . . ."). So I went with them, but not out of zeal to "witness," but to stem my guilt. Those people took a wonderful Christian privilege and made it a mandate, something you must do to stay in God's good graces. They even went so far as to say that one's Christianity was suspect if it didn't include witnessing. Yes, we can even make a law out of spreading the Gospel. And can you imagine how effective our witness is when we do it out of compulsion. I remember speaking to a university colleague about Christ years later. In her youth she had made a profession of faith, but later didn't continue living it out. Her church had drummed into her head that Christianity demanded witnessing. But she didn't feel comfortable nor skillful doing it. It seemed that she was always upsetting her listeners. Imposing that legalism on her resulted in her loss of desire to live the Christian life. She was made to believe that the reality of her faith was conditional to her declaring the gospel to others. You know the old justification game: "You'll want to follow orders (witnessing) if you're a true believer. If not, you're faking it." I empathized with her.

There is no question that Satan loves to see us tamper with such things. In his cunning he twists them for our harm. I experienced his negative influence as I began to give witness of my faith to others, but it took place in quite another way from that of the above examples. I was so zealous to tell of my Christian faith that I often ended up feeling frustrated, bungling and even guilty. I felt inadequate if my listeners didn't put their faith in Christ, especially if they presented arguments I was unable to handle. "If I could just be as sharp as those Christian authors I had read," I said to myself. "They knew how to respond to thorny arguments." Little did I realize that, although those writers presented a number of well thought out controversies and answers, they presented them in writing, which of course always allows for reflection and deliberation. That is different from responding to arguments orally and automatically.

We all have different inadequacies as we talk to others about Christ. There is no need to look in retrospect at our experience by saying, "If only I had said such-and- such." God doesn't send us out to win arguments. Of course it is good to be well-equipped to handle controversies, but that is not the criterion for witnessing. God honors our efforts and uses them in ways beyond imagination. Sometimes we are just seed sowers. Furthermore, we must remember that people have free will either to accept or reject Christ. They may believe in the Savior immediately upon hearing our witness, they may come to Christ later through another person or experience that God brings into their lives, or they may never become Christians.

The point is that their decision is not our responsibility. God never told us *to make Christians*. He simply said to *tell people* about Christ's love. It is out of love for people that we witness to the Good News of Salvation. And that love for humanity is a by-product of our growth in love toward God.

Be that at it may, my grand mistake was that I was fact-oriented. I spoke to others about Christ as if I and they were machines. I didn't have the slightest idea about tenderness, about showing love toward them. I needed to form relationships, without shoving the Bible down their throats. I needed to lighten up, to laugh with them, to accept them where they are, just as Jesus does. But that takes time, something this green, misguided, would-be-evangelist couldn't tolerate. I wanted results, and I wanted them fast. God, we are so stupid. How do you put up with us?

We must also be aware that conversation about religion is becoming increasingly taboo in North American culture. Unlike people in some other countries who enjoy discussion on philosophy, religion, and politics, Americans tend to be uncomfortable talking about such matters, especially their personal views of God. How many times have we heard people say, "Religion is my own business. You are intruding in my personal life."

Ambassadors for Christ

How then do we define our role? The Bible spells it out by declaring us ambassadors for Christ: "as though God were making his appeal through us" (2 Cor. 5:20). Ambassadors are to represent the one who sent them. In that process it is their duty to demonstrate good will in addition to delivering their message. Their personal conduct affects the way the message is received, so they must maintain the highest standards as they approach those to whom they are sent.

Wise ambassadors are sensitive to any sign of displeasure or even anger developing among those to whom they are sent. They are also mindful of the appropriate time for delivering their message. They must take care not to alienate. They show patience. They are kind. They know that their actions will reflect on the message they have been sent to deliver.

Look at Paul's declaration about those who proclaim God's message:

> And the Lord's servant must not quarrel; instead he must be kind to everyone. (2 Tim. 2:24)

Peter adds to that by saying,

> Do this with gentleness and respect. (1 Peter 3:15)

And Jesus said, when giving his lesson about practicing love, that a messenger is no greater than the one who sent him (John 13:16). The courier, then, is to reflect the love of the sender.

Kindness, gentleness, respect, love—key words to keep in mind as we share God's message with others. They carry important signals to our listeners. Christ's ambassadors know that their conduct, when respected, supports the message they are sent to deliver:

> We are therefore Christ's ambassadors, as though God were making his appeal through us. (2 Cor. 5:20)

What an awesome responsibility, yet privilege, we have been given—to offer ourselves as a conduit for God's appeal to others.

Up to now I have discussed witnessing for Christ as a verbal act. There is another way, a more silent one. It is the kind of life we live before others. I have inferred it in the above paragraphs. It can destroy or support our spoken message. Its destructiveness is seen in one's hypocritical actions and attitudes. Its support comes with the evidence we show of our sensitivity toward people.

People whose lives are governed by love can render testimony to God's truth without having to utter a word. How often have we heard someone say, "There's something different about her." Actions often do speak louder than words. What an impact is had by such characteristics as humility, gentleness, kindness, selflessness, and caring. Of course godly living is not an excuse for verbal silence, but it does carry a message that God uses to attract people to him and his ways.

What great things can be accomplished by a person who loves! We are recipients of God's *grace* through *faith* in the Savior, which makes it possible to experience God's *love* for salvation, *love* for him in return, and *love* for people with whom he yearns to fellowship and whom he wishes to bless in ways unimaginable. May our lives reflect his ways so that we may serve others as we faithfully share God's love.

Let's remember that God doesn't present the concept of love as an ideal or mere principle. It is action. Through the Bible he shows us how to activate it in our relations with people. And it will be to their joy, and to our joy too, and especially to God's glory. The Bible contains many directives for Christians to follow. We find ourselves falling short of so many of them—wisdom, knowledge, faith, power, and others we think are critical for doing God's work. They prompt us to fervently pursue God for help in acquiring them. In fact, we often let them dominate us.

They are flashy. They build up our egos. If by chance, however, we should ask God for something entirely different—to help us love people—it will surely prompt God to reply: "Ahhh, you finally understand."

Epilogue

"You have made known to me the paths of life; you will fill me with joy in your presence."

Acts 2:28

I have called attention to a lot of Scripture on grace, faith and love in order to present a biblical rationale for their application to our lives. I realize, however, that the passages cited can be limited to mere knowledge, an accumulation of facts, without applying them to an experiential walk with God. I pray you won't limit yourself in that sort of way.

I have intended this book to be about knowing God, which is for our joy. What I mean by that is knowing him intimately, a knowledge that affects our very being—the way we trust him, wait on him, listen to him, talk to him, rejoice in him, rest in him, and a myriad of other ways which support an attitude that says, "Lord, I see you at work in all aspects of my life, and I love you for it."

The three great words of the Bible I have written about are not for people who are satisfied with their lives, be they

Christian or non-Christian. They are for those who are tired of the way they view life and the way they live it.

For you who may not know Christ for salvation, you can change that by putting your faith in him right now. That is a life-changing experience that Jesus talked about in terms of being born again. You will have God's promise of life eternal and you will become a recipient of his special love and care in all circumstances of your life. It will be the most important step of your life.

For you Christians who want greater joy in walking with God, you have your heavenly Father's provision of grace, faith, and love available for the taking. When you do so, you will become conscious of his involvement in your lives like never before. You will experience the joy of true freedom in Christ: living by grace rather than through your own efforts in following rules; resting in faith instead of worrying and suffering from anxiety; and, loving others in place of thinking solely about yourself. You will find yourself maintaining spiritually healthy behaviors you didn't think yourself capable of. In short, you will leave behind a dull Christian existence in place of a dynamic, fruitful, and satisfying life in Christ. It will be an outcome of great joy for you as well as for those with whom you come in contact.

Your acceptance of his grace through childlike faith will create a bond of intimacy between you and your Heavenly Father resulting in your increased love for him. An awareness of his presence, in fact his living in you, will supplant false notions of a gulf between you and your Creator. It will spur you on to greater communication as you listen to and talk with him. And as you take steps to show God's love in meeting the needs of others—those of fellow saints as well as of those without knowledge of salvation—you will rejoice in the power God gives you as his ambassador. You will be adept in conveying his message with grace, in faith, and with love, because you won't be relying on yourself—your own wisdom and expertise—but on God himself.

Relying on God is the equivalent of allowing him to communicate with us. We let him do that primarily through the Bible. Through that sacred book he teaches many things; however, the instruction can be received as general in nature without making a life-changing impact on us. It needs personalizing if it is to take full effect. Like teaching on the importance of living in accord with humility, or as per gentleness or self-control, we will find his precepts most dynamic when we personalize them; that is, when we relate them to a specific situation in our lives on which we need input. For example, reading about humility, we accept it as a desirable behavior, but it doesn't really hit home until we see a specific circumstance in our lives in which we should be practicing it. Or perhaps it is reading about self-control, which really hits home when we apply it to a given physical problem we are experiencing, like overeating or sexual temptation. Connecting scriptural teaching to our individual lives allows God to communicate in a specific, personalized way. And that engenders intimacy because we see God at work in helping us overcome the negative in our lives.

A word of caution is appropriate here. Don't expect that kind of personalized communication to come about every time you open your Bible. My experience is that God calls things to our attention when he sees us ready to receive them. He knows when we will react positively, when his teaching will be life changing. It may have to do with a multitude of factors at play in our lives that only he understands and capitalizes on when the time is ripe.

God is intimate through other means of communication too, such as through people and circumstances. He often uses people to carry his messages. That is the beauty of care groups—members rendering mutual support as they share messages God lays on their hearts. But then, God's communication through people can go beyond the care group; it can involve any person, a pastor, a friend, or even a stranger, whose speech and/or behavior God uses to call attention to something we need personally. When recognized, it of course becomes life changing for us. The overriding result is that it increases intimacy with God.

Just as God uses people to increase our intimacy with him, so he does through circumstances. God is a master at using any means to communicate to us in a personalized way. He knows our needs, and he works through his creation to fill them. Sometimes we don't become aware of his blessings until years later. Nevertheless, he keeps pouring out his grace, knowing that at some point we will acknowledge his graciousness. It should be a challenge to us to ponder his working each day, and to give him the thanks and praise due him.

A revolution in your life is awaiting as you connect with grace, faith and love. Seize the opportunity! It will result in your experiencing the joy that comes from those wonderful words. Scripture says it this way:

> Peace to the brothers, and *love* with *faith* from God the Father and the Lord Jesus Christ. *Grace* to all who love our Lord Jesus Christ with an undying *love*. (Eph. 6:23–24 emphases mine)

Putting grace, faith and love into practice brings spiritual well-being. Those three great words of the Bible are the ingredients for joyful, abundant living. Grace + Faith + Love = Joy. God's prescriptions for your spiritual health.

Notes

Part I - GRACE

Chapter 1

[1] The scriptural account of the start of the new testament (Matt. 26:28) differs radically from the commonly held idea that the New Testament begins with the Gospel of Matthew. This has profound implications on understanding pre-cross passages that on the surface appear contrary to grace. See Chapter 3 for a discussion on some of these passages.

[2] M. Scott Peck, *Abounding Grace.* (Kansas City: Andrews McMeel, 2000), 137.

[3] Nick Kalivoda, *Heaven's Password.* (Baton Rouge, La: Radio Bible Course), 45.

Part II - FAITH

Chapter 3

[1] Thomas à. Kempis, *The Imitation of Christ*, A Contemporary Version by William Griffin. (New York: HarperCollins, 2000), 6.

[2] For an analysis of the misapplication of Scripture about health and wealth, see Ken L. Sarles, "A Theological Evaluation of the Prosperity Gospel," in *Bibliotheca Sacra* (Oct-Dec., 1986).

Part III - LOVE

Chapter 4

[1] C. S. Lewis, *The Four Loves,* (New York: Harcourt, Brace, 1960), 13.

[2] A. W. Tozer, *The Pursuit of God,* (Old Tappan, New Jersey: Fleming H. Revell, 1948).

Chapter 5

[1] G. K. Chesterton, 1985. *As I Was Saying*, (Grand Rapids, Michigan: Erdmans, 1985), 267.

[2] Ibid.

[3] We should be aware that those early believers met for the express purpose of encouraging, exhorting and edifying one another. Unfortunately the Corinthians did it with disorder, in the form of rude interruptions. It was so blatant a disregard for civility that it causes us to focus on the disorder rather than on the original intent of the gathering. That intent becomes obvious as we see them sharing mutually. Yes, they were disorderly, and they are not to be excused for it, but they knew the importance of each member participating actively. Note that Paul didn't tell them to stop mutual strengthening. He didn't tell them to let one person do it all. It was God's design for Christians to assume responsibility to care for one another. That means everybody participating.

[4] Singing may become a part of the meeting's function if a time of worship is to be set aside as part of the agenda. I have found singing more meaningful when done without

hymnbooks, because the absence of printed words and notes allows for greater concentration on the spiritual message of the songs. It also provides for singing prayerfully, even with eyes closed, to enhance concentration and personal communication with the Lord. It reduces superficial mouthing of lyrics, of which we are all sometimes guilty. Singing without books, however, requires familiarity with the hymns' melodies and words, which some participants may lack. But this can be overcome over time as group members learn the hymns and choruses that are most frequently sung. Until this stage is reached, however, hymnbooks may constitute a necessary tool.

[5] There is much to be said for prayer requests involving one's own life rather than the lives of others. Most often prayers in church meetings pertain to other people. For example, "pray for my neighbor's cousin," which shows a healthy concern for friends and relatives. But don't participants have needs of their own? Openness in declaring *our* needs is an important part of making prayer requests in the care group

About the Author

Dr. Kalivoda utilizes his years of biblical study and personal experience to challenge readers to embrace grace, faith and love as the means of establishing a dynamic, intimate relationship with God. He has experienced the joys of biblical Christianity as well as the sorrows of scriptural misinterpretation and people-designed religion. He calls on readers to take a fresh look at how God wants them to experience the joy of practicing grace, faith and love in place of holding to mere cognitive understanding of those words.

The author served as professor and administrator at three major universities: Louisiana State University, as Director of Latin American Relations and Coordinator of the LSU Caribbean Armed Forces Program in the Panama Canal Zone; Oklahoma State University, as International Student Advisor and Assistant Professor of Spanish; and, the University of Georgia, as Professor of Foreign Language Education, Spanish, and Chairman of the American Language Program, where he distinguished himself in research and publication in the field of language acquisition and teaching.

Dr. Kalivoda has published over 50 articles, monographs, and books on language learning and pedagogy, and has been a popular speaker at national and international conferences. He has been honored with several national awards.

He and his wife Deleta live in St. Charles, Missouri, where they are active in lay ministries.

To order additional copies of

Great Words of the Bible

Prescriptions for Spiritual Health

Have your credit card ready and call:

1-877-421-READ (7323)

or please visit our web site at
www.pleasantword.com

Also available at: www.amazon.com

Printed in the United States
24444LVS00001B/235-243

9 781414 100555